Mind Over Matter
The Science of Self-Healing

Introduction to Self-Healing

In an age where the pace of life quickens with every passing moment, the pursuit of health and well-being has become paramount. Yet, amidst the myriad of modern medical advancements and health trends, lies an ancient, yet profoundly relevant concept: self-healing. This book, "Mind Over Matter: The Science of Self-Healing," is an invitation to explore the remarkable capacity of the human body and mind to heal itself. It's a journey through the intricate connections between the mind, body, and spirit, illuminated by science, enriched by practice, and brought to life through stories of transformation.

Self-healing is not a replacement for professional medical advice or treatment; rather, it's a complement, a forgotten dimension of our inherent nature that when rediscovered, can enhance our health, vitality, and quality of life. This book aims to demystify the principles of self-healing, presenting them in a way that is accessible, engaging, and actionable. Whether you are navigating a health challenge, seeking to optimize your well-being, or simply curious about the untapped powers within you, this book offers insights, techniques, and inspiration.

The Evolution of Self-Healing Concepts

The concept of self-healing is as old as humanity itself, rooted in the earliest civilizations and healing traditions around the world. From the shamans of tribal cultures to the physicians of ancient Greece, the ability of the body to heal itself has always been recognized, albeit understood in vastly different ways through the ages.

In ancient times, healing was often viewed holistically, with an emphasis on the balance between the physical, mental, and spiritual aspects of a person. Treatments were not only aimed at alleviating physical symptoms but also at restoring this balance, using a variety of methods from herbal remedies to meditation and ritual.

As medical science advanced, particularly in the West, the focus shifted towards a more reductionist approach, emphasizing the treatment of specific ailments through medical interventions and pharmaceuticals. This shift brought about remarkable advancements in acute care and the management of diseases but often at the expense of recognizing the body's innate ability to heal and the role of the mind and emotions in this process.

In recent decades, however, there has been a resurgence of interest in the holistic approach to health and healing. This renewed interest is fueled by a growing body of scientific research that underscores the profound connection between the mind and body and the tangible effects of mental and emotional states on physical health. Practices such as mindfulness, meditation, and visualization, once considered fringe or alternative, are now being recognized for their therapeutic potential, backed by evidence of their benefits.

This book traces the arc of self-healing concepts from their ancient roots to their modern incarnations, weaving together the wisdom of the past with the scientific discoveries of today. It's a testament to the timeless nature of the human quest for health and wholeness, and a guide for harnessing the incredible potential that lies within each of us.

As we embark on this exploration, remember that self-healing is not a one-size-fits-all proposition. It's a personal journey, unique to each individual. My hope is that you will find within these pages not only valuable information but also inspiration to experiment, to explore, and to embrace the possibilities of self-healing in your own life.

Why This Matters Now

In an era marked by unprecedented technological advancements, soaring healthcare costs, and a global health landscape challenged by chronic diseases and mental health crises, the relevance of self-healing has never been more pronounced. This section delves into the reasons why the principles and practices of self-healing are not just beneficial but essential in our contemporary context.

The Healthcare Paradox

Despite remarkable progress in medical science, many societies face a healthcare paradox: increasing healthcare expenditure does not necessarily correlate with better health outcomes. Chronic diseases such as diabetes, heart disease, and mental health disorders are on the rise, often exacerbated by lifestyle factors that conventional healthcare models are ill-equipped to address comprehensively. Self-healing offers a complementary path, emphasizing prevention, holistic well-being, and the individual's active role in their health journey.

The Rise of Mental Health Awareness

Mental health has emerged from the shadows to become a central theme in discussions about health and well-being. The recognition of mental health's critical role in overall health underscores the need for approaches that transcend medication and therapy. Self-healing practices such as mindfulness, meditation, and emotional regulation offer valuable tools for managing stress, anxiety, and depression, contributing to a more holistic approach to mental wellness.

The Empowerment Movement

There is a growing movement towards personal empowerment in health and well-being. People increasingly seek to take control of their health, armed with information from a variety of sources. Self-healing represents a pivotal aspect of this movement, offering individuals the knowledge and tools to influence their health outcomes positively. It champions the idea that while professional medical advice is indispensable, individuals also possess the power to effect change within their bodies and minds.

The Integration of Traditional Wisdom and Modern Science

Today's interest in self-healing also signifies a bridging of the gap between ancient healing wisdom and contemporary scientific understanding. Practices once considered purely spiritual or anecdotal are now being studied and validated by scientific research. This convergence is fostering a more integrative approach to health, where traditional wisdom and modern science collaborate to enhance human well-being.

The Quest for Quality of Life

Ultimately, the resurgence of self-healing reflects a collective quest for not just longer life but improved quality of life. In a world where life expectancy has increased, individuals aspire to live those extra years with vitality, purpose, and well-being. Self-healing practices offer pathways to achieve this, emphasizing the quality of life as much as its quantity.

Why This Matters Now encapsulates a timely response to the complexities of modern health challenges. It acknowledges the limitations of existing healthcare paradigms and proposes self-healing as a vital supplement to traditional medical care. By empowering individuals with the knowledge and tools to engage in their healing process, self-healing practices promise not only to alleviate physical and mental ailments but also to enrich lives with a deeper sense of wellness and fulfillment. As we navigate the pressures and possibilities of the 21st century, the principles of self-healing invite us to rediscover the profound connections between mind, body, and spirit, offering hope and direction for a healthier, more harmonious world.

Chapter 1: Understanding the Mind-Body Connection

Historical Perspectives

The exploration of the mind-body connection is not a new endeavor; it is a journey that humanity has embarked upon for millennia. This profound relationship between our mental states and physical health has been a cornerstone of medical philosophies and practices across various cultures and epochs. Understanding this connection requires us to look back at the wisdom of ancient civilizations, where the seeds of today's knowledge were first sown.

Historically, the concept of a mind-body connection was inherent to the holistic view of health. Ancient healing traditions did not make a strict distinction between the mind and the body, viewing them instead as parts of a unified whole. This perspective is evident in the healing practices of civilizations such as the Egyptians, Greeks, Chinese, and Indians, each of which contributed uniquely to the development of this concept.

Ancient Wisdom and Practices

Egyptian Civilization: In ancient Egypt, health was believed to be the result of a balance between physical, emotional, and spiritual aspects of life. The Egyptians practiced a form of medicine that incorporated magical and religious rituals alongside physical treatments, reflecting an understanding of the mind-body-spirit triad.

Greek Medicine: Perhaps no ancient culture has influenced Western medicine as much as the Greeks, with Hippocrates often hailed as the "Father of Medicine." Hippocrates introduced the idea that disease was a result of natural causes and not merely the wrath of the gods. He emphasized the importance of diet, environment, and lifestyle on health, laying the groundwork for the mind-body connection in medicine.

Chinese Medicine: Traditional Chinese Medicine (TCM) has a rich history of understanding the mind-body connection, with its foundations in the concept of Qi (vital energy) and the balance of Yin and Yang. Practices such as acupuncture, tai chi, and qigong are based on the belief that health is achieved by harmonizing the body's energy flow, demonstrating an intricate link between the physical body and mental state.

Indian Ayurveda: Ayurveda, the traditional system of medicine in India, is built on the premise that life represents a balance between the body, mind, soul, and senses. It prescribes a personalized approach to health, emphasizing diet, herbal remedies, meditation, yoga, and physical exercise to maintain or restore this balance, highlighting the interdependence of mind and body.

These ancient practices were not merely medical treatments but philosophies of living that integrated physical health, mental well-being, and spiritual development. They recognized that emotions and thoughts could manifest physically, affecting health and that, conversely, physical conditions could influence mental states.

The wisdom of these ancients, though sometimes overlooked or dismissed by later scientific developments, has endured and is being revisited in the light of contemporary research. Today, as we delve deeper into the mechanisms of the mind-body connection through the lens of modern science, we find echoes of these ancient insights, reaffirming the timeless truth that health is a holistic state encompassing the mind, body, and spirit. This chapter seeks to bridge the ancient with the modern, illustrating how historical perspectives on the mind-body connection are being validated and expanded upon in today's scientific and medical communities.

The Renaissance of Mind-Body Medicine

The resurgence of interest in the mind-body connection, often referred to as the Renaissance of Mind-Body Medicine, marks a pivotal shift in contemporary healthcare and wellness paradigms. This movement, gaining momentum in the late 20th and early 21st centuries, is characterized by a growing recognition of the integral role that mental, emotional, and spiritual well-being plays in physical health. This section explores the factors contributing to this renaissance and its implications for modern medicine and individual wellness.

Integrating Eastern and Western Philosophies

One of the key drivers of the mind-body medicine renaissance has been the integration of Eastern healing philosophies with Western medical practices. As globalization facilitated cross-cultural exchanges, Western societies became increasingly aware of Eastern practices such as meditation, yoga, and traditional Chinese medicine. Scientific research began to validate the health benefits of these practices, offering a compelling evidence base that bridged ancient wisdom with modern science.

Advancements in Psychoneuroimmunology

The field of psychoneuroimmunology (PNI) has played a significant role in the renaissance of mind-body medicine. PNI studies the complex interactions between the nervous system, the endocrine system, and the immune system, and how these interactions are influenced by psychological processes. Research in this field has provided concrete evidence of how stress, emotions, and thought patterns can directly affect immune function, hormone levels, and overall physical health. These findings have underscored the scientific validity of the mind-body connection, encouraging a more holistic approach to health and disease management.

The Holistic Health Movement

Parallel to scientific advancements, there has been a growing consumer demand for a more holistic approach to health. This movement emphasizes the importance of treating the whole person rather than just the symptoms of disease. It advocates for preventative healthcare measures, lifestyle changes, and natural remedies, alongside conventional medical treatments. The holistic health movement has propelled the popularity of mind-body practices and has pushed the healthcare industry to adopt more integrative approaches to treatment and wellness.

Technological Innovations

Technological innovations have also played a part in the resurgence of mind-body medicine. Wearable devices, mobile apps, and virtual platforms have made mind-body practices more accessible to the general public. They offer guided meditations, stress management tools, and biofeedback mechanisms that allow individuals to actively engage in their health and well-being. These technologies have not only democratized access to mind-body practices but have also contributed to their normalization and acceptance in daily life.

The Rise of Personal Empowerment

Finally, the renaissance of mind-body medicine reflects a broader cultural shift towards personal empowerment in health. With more information and tools at their disposal, individuals are taking greater responsibility for their health outcomes. There is a growing recognition that health is not merely the absence of disease but a state of complete physical, mental, and social well-being, as defined by the World Health Organization. This perspective empowers individuals to explore and incorporate mind-body practices as essential components of their health and wellness routines.

The renaissance of mind-body medicine represents a convergence of historical wisdom, scientific validation, and cultural evolution. It is a testament to the enduring relevance of the mind-body connection and its potential to transform our approach to health and healing. As we continue to explore and understand this connection, we open the door to more compassionate, comprehensive, and effective healthcare practices that honor the whole person.

Modern Scientific Research

In recent decades, the exploration of the mind-body connection has transitioned from philosophical speculation to empirical investigation, thanks to advances in modern scientific research. This body of work encompasses a wide range of disciplines, including neuroscience, psychology, medicine, and genetics, among others. Through rigorous study, scientists have begun to unravel the intricate mechanisms through which the mind influences physical health, and vice versa, providing a robust foundation for the principles of mind-body medicine.

Key Studies and Findings

The Impact of Stress on Physical Health

One of the most significant areas of research in mind-body medicine is the study of stress and its physiological effects. Seminal studies by researchers such as Robert Sapolsky have shown how chronic stress can lead to or exacerbate health problems by triggering the body's "fight or flight" response, leading to elevated levels of cortisol and adrenaline. These hormones, while beneficial in short bursts, can cause long-term damage when consistently elevated, contributing to heart disease, hypertension, and a weakened immune response.

Mindfulness and Meditation

Research on mindfulness and meditation has provided compelling evidence of their benefits on physical and mental health. Studies have shown that regular meditation practice can lead to reductions in stress, anxiety, and depression, as well as improvements in pain tolerance, immune function, and cardiovascular health. Neuroimaging studies have even demonstrated that meditation can lead to structural changes in the brain, including increased grey matter density in areas associated with attention, emotional regulation, and self-awareness.

The Placebo Effect

The placebo effect serves as a fascinating example of the mind's capacity to influence physical healing. Research has demonstrated that the belief in the effectiveness of a harmless substance or procedure can lead to real physiological improvements in health. This effect underscores the power of expectation and belief in the healing process, suggesting that the mind's positive convictions can significantly contribute to treatment outcomes.

Biofeedback and Neurofeedback

Studies on biofeedback and neurofeedback have shown how individuals can learn to control physiological processes that are typically considered involuntary, such as heart rate, blood pressure, and brain wave patterns. This research illustrates the potential for individuals to actively participate in their own healing processes through increased self-awareness and control over their bodily functions.

Psychoneuroimmunology (PNI)

PNI research has provided insights into how psychological factors can affect the immune system. For example, studies have found that stress, depression, and social isolation can negatively impact immune response, while positive emotions and social support can enhance it. This area of research highlights the complex interplay between the nervous system, endocrine system, and immune system, mediated by psychological states.

Epigenetics and the Mind-Body Connection

Emerging research in the field of epigenetics has revealed how lifestyle and environmental factors, including mental and emotional states, can influence gene expression. This research suggests that positive interventions such as stress reduction, healthy social interactions, and mindfulness practices can lead to epigenetic changes that promote health and well-being.

These key studies and findings represent just a fraction of the extensive research supporting the mind-body connection. Together, they provide a scientific basis for the efficacy of mind-body practices and underscore the potential for integrative approaches to health and healing. As the body of evidence continues to grow, it paves the way for new treatments and therapies that harness the power of the mind to influence physical health, offering hope and healing to those seeking a more holistic approach to well-being.

Neuroscientific Perspectives

The field of neuroscience has significantly advanced our understanding of the mind-body connection, offering insights into how the brain communicates with the rest of the body and influences overall health. Neuroscientific research has illuminated the pathways through which thoughts, emotions, and mental states can affect physical well-being, providing a biological basis for the impact of mental processes on health.

Brain-Body Communication

Central to the neuroscientific perspective is the concept of brain-body communication, which occurs through a complex network of neural, hormonal, and immunological pathways. The brain sends and receives signals to and from the body via the nervous system, influencing physiological responses and modulating functions such as stress response, immune function, and pain perception. This bidirectional communication underscores the interconnectedness of mental states and physical health.

The Role of the Autonomic Nervous System

The autonomic nervous system (ANS) plays a crucial role in this communication, regulating involuntary bodily functions such as heart rate, digestion, and respiratory rate. The ANS consists of two main branches: the sympathetic nervous system (SNS), which mobilizes the body's resources in response to stress or threat, and the parasympathetic nervous system (PNS), which promotes relaxation and healing. Neuroscientific research has shown how practices that induce relaxation, such as meditation and deep-breathing exercises, can activate the PNS, counteracting the stress-induced activities of the SNS and promoting health and well-being.

Neuroplasticity and Healing

Another key concept in the neuroscientific perspective is neuroplasticity—the brain's ability to reorganize itself by forming new neural connections throughout life. This adaptability is crucial for learning and memory and plays a significant role in recovery from brain injury and coping with stress. Mind-body practices like meditation, mindfulness, and cognitive-behavioral therapy can enhance neuroplasticity, leading to improved emotional regulation, reduced symptoms of anxiety and depression, and better stress management.

The Endocrine System and Stress Response

Neuroscience has also shed light on the relationship between the brain and the endocrine system, particularly in the context of the stress response. The hypothalamic-pituitary-adrenal (HPA) axis is a key component of this relationship, with the brain's perception of stress triggering a hormonal cascade that results in the release of cortisol and other stress hormones. Chronic activation of the HPA axis can lead to a range of health issues, including anxiety disorders, depression, and cardiovascular disease. Research into stress reduction techniques has shown potential for mitigating these effects by modulating the activity of the HPA axis.

Pain Perception and Management

Finally, neuroscientific research into pain perception has provided valuable insights into the mind-body connection. The experience of pain is not solely the result of physical injury but is also influenced by psychological factors such as attention, mood, and expectations. Techniques that alter the mental processing of pain, such as mindfulness-based stress reduction (MBSR) and cognitive-behavioral therapy (CBT), have been shown to be effective in managing chronic pain by changing the way pain is perceived and processed in the brain.

In conclusion, neuroscientific perspectives on the mind-body connection highlight the powerful influence of the brain on physical health. By elucidating the mechanisms through which mental states affect bodily functions, neuroscience supports the integration of mind-body practices into health care, offering promising avenues for enhancing health and treating disease. This research underscores the importance of a holistic approach to health that acknowledges the interplay between the mind and the body.

Case Studies

The exploration of the mind-body connection through case studies, particularly those involving remarkable recoveries, provides compelling evidence of the powerful interplay between mental states and physical health. These stories not only inspire but also offer valuable insights into the potential for self-healing and the impact of psychological factors on overcoming illness.

Case Study 1: Overcoming Chronic Pain through Mindfulness

One significant case involves a patient suffering from chronic pain for over a decade, resulting from a severe car accident. Traditional medical treatments had little effect, and the patient's quality of life was significantly diminished. The turning point came when the patient began a program of Mindfulness-Based Stress Reduction (MBSR). Through consistent practice, the patient learned to change their relationship with pain, focusing on acceptance and mindful awareness rather than resistance. Remarkably, within months, the patient reported a significant reduction in pain levels and an improvement in overall well-being. This case highlights the potential of mindfulness to modulate pain perception and emphasizes the brain's role in pain management.

Case Study 2: Healing from Autoimmune Disease with Lifestyle Changes

Another inspiring story involves an individual diagnosed with an autoimmune disease, which conventional medicine deemed incurable. Facing a lifetime of medication and its side effects, the patient sought alternative approaches. By radically changing their diet, incorporating regular yoga and meditation practices, and adopting stress reduction techniques, the patient experienced a dramatic improvement in symptoms. Medical tests eventually revealed a significant reduction in autoimmune markers. This case illustrates the potential for lifestyle interventions to influence the course of chronic diseases and underscores the importance of a holistic approach to health.

Case Study 3: Recovering from Depression through Exercise and Social Support

A notable case of mental health recovery involves an individual suffering from severe depression, unresponsive to medication and therapy. As a complementary approach, the patient was encouraged to engage in regular aerobic exercise and to participate in community support groups. Over time, the patient reported improvements in mood, energy levels, and outlook on life. The exercise acted not only as a natural antidepressant but also enhanced the patient's sense of social connection and support. This case demonstrates the interconnection between physical activity, social well-being, and mental health, offering a model for integrative mental health care.

Case Study 4: Heart Disease Reversed with Comprehensive Lifestyle Changes

A groundbreaking case study by Dr. Dean Ornish showed that patients with coronary heart disease could actually reverse their condition through comprehensive lifestyle changes, without reliance on surgery or medication. These changes included a plant-based diet, regular physical activity, stress management techniques (including meditation and yoga), and strong social support. Follow-up tests showed not only a halt in the progression of the disease but actual reversal of arterial blockage. This case provides strong evidence for the power of lifestyle medicine and the potential for self-healing even in the face of serious physical illnesses.

Case Study 5: Cancer Patients and Visualization Techniques

Finally, there are documented cases of cancer patients who, alongside conventional treatments, employed visualization techniques to imagine their bodies fighting off cancer cells. Some of these patients showed remarkable recoveries, with researchers speculating that such mental exercises might boost the immune system or create a more positive and hopeful mindset, which in turn could contribute to physical healing. While not a standalone treatment, this approach exemplifies the potential synergy between mind and body in the healing process.

These case studies, drawn from a range of conditions and approaches, underscore the complex and dynamic relationship between the mind and body. They highlight the potential of integrative, holistic approaches to health and recovery, suggesting that empowering patients with mind-body practices can be a valuable complement to conventional medical treatment. The remarkable recoveries documented in these cases serve as a testament to the healing potential inherent within each individual, reinforcing the importance of exploring and understanding the mind-body connection.

Analysis and Insights

The case studies of remarkable recoveries provide not only inspiration but also critical insights into the dynamics of the mind-body connection. Through analysis of these cases, several key themes and insights emerge, offering valuable lessons for both individuals seeking health and wellness and the broader medical community.

The Power of the Mind in Physical Healing

One of the most striking insights is the influential role of mental and emotional states in physical healing. Whether it's through mindfulness, visualization, or positive thinking, the cases demonstrate how mental activities can significantly impact physiological processes. This connection suggests that fostering a positive, hopeful mindset could be a crucial component of any treatment plan.

Holistic Approach to Health

The cases also reinforce the importance of a holistic approach to health, where mental, emotional, and lifestyle factors are considered alongside physical symptoms. This approach acknowledges the complex interplay of various elements of health and emphasizes the need for comprehensive treatment plans that address all aspects of a person's well-being.

Individualized Treatment

Another insight is the significance of individualized treatment. Each case study presents a unique combination of methods and practices tailored to the individual's specific needs, preferences, and circumstances. This customization underscores the idea that there is no one-size-fits-all solution in health and healing, and treatment plans should be as unique as the individuals they are designed for.

The Role of Lifestyle Changes

The case studies also highlight the profound impact of lifestyle changes on health. Dietary modifications, exercise, stress reduction, and social support are recurring themes in these stories of recovery. These factors not only contribute to the prevention and management of various health conditions but can also play a role in reversing them.

Integrating Conventional and Alternative Medicine

Importantly, these case studies illustrate the potential benefits of integrating conventional medical treatments with alternative and complementary approaches. This integration allows for a more comprehensive treatment strategy, harnessing the strengths of both conventional medicine (such as its effectiveness in acute care and disease management) and alternative practices (such as their focus on prevention and holistic care).

Empowering Patients

Finally, a crucial insight from these case studies is the empowerment of patients in their healing journey. By actively participating in their health through self-care practices, lifestyle choices, and mind-body techniques, patients can take an active role in their healing process, which can lead to better health outcomes and a greater sense of control over their well-being.

In conclusion, the analysis of these case studies of remarkable recoveries provides valuable lessons in understanding and utilizing the mind-body connection for health and healing. It underscores the need for a more integrated, holistic, and personalized approach to healthcare, where patients are empowered to play an active role in their health and well-being. These insights pave the way for a more comprehensive and compassionate approach to medicine, one that fully embraces the intricate interplay between the mind and the body.

Chapter 2: The Psychology of Healing

The Role of Beliefs and Attitudes

Understanding the psychology of healing requires delving into the foundational role that beliefs and attitudes play in health and recovery. The mind's power to influence physical well-being is profound, with an individual's mindset often serving as a catalyst for healing or, conversely, as a barrier to it. This section explores how beliefs and attitudes impact the healing process, drawing on psychological theories, research findings, and practical applications.

The Impact of Beliefs on Health Outcomes

Beliefs about health, illness, and healing can significantly affect health outcomes. Positive beliefs and expectations can enhance the body's healing responses, a phenomenon observed in the placebo effect, where patients experience real improvements in health outcomes based on their belief in the effectiveness of a treatment, even if the treatment is inert. Conversely, negative beliefs and attitudes, such as hopelessness or pessimism, can impede recovery and exacerbate health conditions, a phenomenon known as the nocebo effect.

Mindset and Recovery

The concept of mindset—whether fixed or growth-oriented—also plays a critical role in the healing process. A growth mindset, characterized by the belief in the ability to change and improve one's condition through effort and perseverance, has been linked to better health outcomes. This mindset encourages resilience, adaptive coping strategies, and a proactive approach to healing, facilitating recovery and well-being.

Self-Efficacy in Healing

Self-efficacy, or the belief in one's ability to influence outcomes in one's life, is another critical factor in the psychology of healing. High levels of self-efficacy are associated with increased motivation to take charge of one's health, engage in healthy behaviors, and adhere to treatment regimens. This belief in personal agency supports active participation in the healing process, leading to more positive health outcomes.

The Role of Attitudes Toward Illness and Treatment

Attitudes toward illness and treatment—whether optimistic, realistic, or pessimistic—can significantly influence how individuals cope with health challenges. An optimistic attitude, while maintaining realism about the condition and its challenges, can foster resilience and a positive outlook, enhancing the effectiveness of treatments and the overall healing process.

In contrast, negative attitudes can lead to decreased motivation, poor adherence to treatment plans, and worsened health outcomes.

Cultural Beliefs and Healing

Cultural beliefs and practices also profoundly impact the healing process. Different cultures have unique perspectives on health, illness, and healing, influencing individuals' attitudes toward medical treatment, alternative therapies, and the healing process itself. Understanding and respecting these cultural differences is crucial in providing effective, holistic care that aligns with patients' values and beliefs.

Harnessing Beliefs and Attitudes for Healing

Recognizing the power of beliefs and attitudes in the healing process opens avenues for interventions designed to foster positive mindsets and enhance recovery. Techniques such as cognitive-behavioral therapy (CBT), mindfulness-based stress reduction (MBSR), and motivational interviewing can help individuals cultivate more positive, health-promoting beliefs and attitudes. These interventions can empower patients, enabling them to play an active role in their healing journey, and underscore the importance of addressing the psychological dimensions of health as part of a comprehensive approach to care.

In conclusion, the role of beliefs and attitudes in the psychology of healing is both profound and multifaceted. By understanding and leveraging this aspect of the mind-body connection, individuals and healthcare providers can enhance the effectiveness of medical treatments and support the body's natural healing processes, leading to improved health outcomes and well-being.

The Placebo Effect

The placebo effect stands as a compelling demonstration of the mind's capacity to influence physical health, encapsulating the profound interplay between psychological factors and biological responses. This phenomenon occurs when an inactive substance or sham treatment triggers a real, positive change in a patient's medical condition, purely based on the individual's expectation of benefit. The placebo effect underscores the power of beliefs and attitudes in the healing process and offers valuable insights into the psychology of healing.

Understanding the Placebo Effect

At its core, the placebo effect is rooted in perception and expectation. When patients believe they are receiving an effective treatment, their bodies can initiate physiological changes that mimic those produced by actual medical treatments. This effect can manifest in various ways, including pain relief, improved motor function, and alleviation of symptoms in conditions ranging from depression to Parkinson's disease.

Mechanisms Behind the Placebo Effect

The mechanisms underlying the placebo effect are complex and multifaceted, involving a combination of psychological and neurobiological processes. Research has shown that the placebo effect can activate the brain's reward pathways and release endogenous opioids, natural painkillers that mimic the effect of drugs like morphine. Additionally, placebos can modulate brain activity in regions associated with mood, pain perception, and stress response, further contributing to their therapeutic effects.

Factors Influencing the Placebo Effect

Several factors can influence the magnitude and likelihood of the placebo effect, including:

- Patient Expectations: The stronger a patient's expectation of benefit, the more pronounced the placebo effect can be. These expectations can be shaped by previous experiences, the perceived credibility of the treatment, and the manner in which the treatment is presented.
- The Doctor-Patient Relationship: The quality of the interaction between healthcare providers and patients can significantly impact the placebo effect. A supportive, empathetic approach can enhance patients' expectations of treatment efficacy, thereby amplifying the placebo response.
- The Context of Treatment: The environment and context in which treatment is administered also play a role. Treatments administered in what are perceived as high-tech or professional medical settings may elicit a stronger placebo response than those given in less formal environments.

Implications for Clinical Practice

The placebo effect has important implications for clinical practice and medical research. It highlights the necessity of using placebo controls in clinical trials to accurately assess the efficacy of new treatments. Moreover, the placebo effect underscores the importance of considering psychological and contextual factors in patient care. By recognizing and harnessing the power of the placebo effect, healthcare providers can enhance the therapeutic impact of treatments, even when the effect is not solely attributable to the active ingredients of the treatment itself.

Ethical Considerations

While the placebo effect can be beneficial, it also raises ethical questions, particularly regarding transparency and informed consent. It is crucial to balance the potential benefits of the placebo effect with the need to maintain patients' trust and ensure that they are fully informed about their treatment options.

In conclusion, the placebo effect vividly illustrates the significant role of the mind in healing and the importance of psychological factors in medical treatment. By deepening our understanding of this phenomenon, we can better appreciate the complex interplay between mind and body and explore new ways to optimize health and healing.

Shifting Mindsets for Healing

The concept of shifting mindsets for healing delves into the transformative power of altering one's mental approach and attitude towards health, illness, and recovery. This shift in perspective is not just about positive thinking but involves a deeper change in how individuals perceive their ability to influence their health outcomes. Embracing a mindset geared towards growth, resilience, and empowerment can significantly impact one's journey to healing and well-being.

Understanding Mindset Shifts

A mindset shift in the context of healing involves moving from a passive to an active role in one's health journey. It encompasses:

- From Fixed to Growth: Transitioning from a fixed mindset, where one believes their health and abilities are static and unchangeable, to a growth mindset, where one sees potential for improvement and healing through effort and strategy.
- From Victim to Empowered: Shifting from seeing oneself as a victim of circumstance or illness to embracing a sense of empowerment, recognizing the ability to make choices and take actions that positively impact health.
- From Isolation to Connection: Moving from a sense of isolation in one's health challenges to seeking and valuing connection with others, understanding that support networks play a crucial role in the healing process.

The Role of Self-Compassion

Shifting mindsets for healing also involves cultivating self-compassion. Recognizing and accepting one's suffering with kindness rather than judgment can alleviate emotional distress and promote a more supportive internal environment for healing. Self-compassion encourages resilience, making it easier to cope with health challenges and engage in positive health behaviors.

Strategies for Shifting Mindsets

1. Cognitive Reframing: This involves identifying and challenging negative or limiting beliefs about one's health and replacing them with more positive, empowering thoughts. It's about seeing challenges as opportunities for growth and learning.

2. Mindfulness and Meditation: These practices can help individuals become more aware of their thoughts and feelings without judgment, fostering a shift towards acceptance and presence. This awareness can be pivotal in changing one's relationship with pain, stress, and illness.

3. Goal Setting and Visualization: Setting realistic, achievable goals and visualizing positive outcomes can reinforce a growth mindset. Visualization can be particularly powerful, as imagining oneself successfully managing health challenges can enhance motivation and confidence.

4. Seeking Support: Engaging with supportive communities, whether through therapy, support groups, or with friends and family, can foster a sense of connection and shared experience. Such support can validate feelings and provide encouragement for mindset shifts.

Impact on Health Outcomes

Research and anecdotal evidence suggest that shifting mindsets can lead to improved health outcomes. Individuals who adopt a more empowered, growth-oriented approach to their health often report higher levels of satisfaction with life, better mental health, and, in some cases, improved physical health markers. These benefits are attributed to increased engagement in healthy behaviors, improved stress management, and a greater sense of control over one's health.

Challenges and Considerations

While shifting mindsets for healing offers many benefits, it's important to recognize the challenges. Deep-seated beliefs and patterns of thinking can be difficult to change, requiring time, patience, and persistence. Additionally, mindset shifts should not be seen as a panacea; they are most effective when combined with conventional medical treatments and healthy lifestyle choices.

In conclusion, shifting mindsets for healing represents a powerful tool in the journey towards health and well-being. By fostering a growth mindset, cultivating self-compassion, and embracing empowerment, individuals can significantly influence their path to recovery and overall quality of life. This approach underscores the importance of integrating psychological well-being with physical health, offering a more holistic view of healing.

Stress and Its Impact on Health

Stress, a universal human experience, plays a significant role in health and disease. Its impact on physical and mental well-being is profound and wide-ranging, affecting everything from the immune system to mental health, cardiovascular health, and beyond. Understanding the mechanisms through which stress influences health, as well as strategies to mitigate its effects, is crucial for promoting overall well-being.

Understanding Stress

Stress is the body's response to any demand or challenge. When faced with a stressor, the body reacts with a "fight-or-flight" response, activating the nervous system and releasing stress hormones like cortisol and adrenaline. This response is crucial for survival, preparing the body to react quickly to dangerous situations. However, when activated too frequently or for too long, it can lead to health problems.

The Biological Impact of Stress

- Immune System: Chronic stress can suppress the immune system, making the body more susceptible to infections and slowing down wound healing. It can also exacerbate autoimmune diseases.
- Cardiovascular System: Stress increases heart rate and blood pressure, strains the heart, and elevates levels of cholesterol and triglycerides, contributing to the buildup of plaque in arteries (atherosclerosis) and increasing the risk of heart attack and stroke.

- Mental Health: Stress is a known risk factor for mental health disorders, including depression and anxiety. It can also lead to stress-related disorders such as post-traumatic stress disorder (PTSD).
- Digestive System: Stress can affect the gut-brain axis, leading to or exacerbating gastrointestinal problems like gastroesophageal reflux disease (GERD), peptic ulcer disease, irritable bowel syndrome (IBS), and more.
- Endocrine System: Chronic stress can lead to dysregulation of the hypothalamic-pituitary-adrenal (HPA) axis, affecting hormones that regulate metabolism, immune function, and other vital processes.

Psychological and Behavioral Effects

Stress not only has direct physiological effects but also influences behavior, which can further impact health. Under stress, individuals may adopt unhealthy behaviors such as smoking, excessive alcohol consumption, overeating, or physical inactivity. These behaviors, in turn, increase the risk of numerous health conditions, including obesity, type 2 diabetes, and substance use disorders.

Managing and Reducing Stress

Reducing stress and its impact on health involves both managing the source of stress and enhancing the body's ability to cope. Strategies include:

- Lifestyle Changes: Regular physical activity, a balanced diet, sufficient sleep, and limiting alcohol and caffeine intake can help reduce stress levels and improve overall health.
- Mindfulness and Relaxation Techniques: Practices such as meditation, yoga, deep breathing exercises, and progressive muscle relaxation can activate the body's relaxation response, counteracting the effects of stress.
- Social Support: Building and maintaining strong relationships with friends, family, and community can provide emotional support and reduce the psychological impact of stress.
- Professional Help: When stress becomes overwhelming or chronic, seeking the assistance of a psychologist or counselor can provide strategies to manage stress effectively, including cognitive-behavioral therapy (CBT) and other forms of psychological support.

The Importance of Addressing Stress

Recognizing and addressing stress is vital for preventing its detrimental effects on health. By adopting a holistic approach to stress management that includes lifestyle modifications, psychological strategies, and social support, individuals can enhance their resilience to stress and improve their overall well-being. In doing so, it is possible to mitigate the diverse and far-reaching impacts of stress on health, leading to a healthier, more balanced life.

The Biology of Stress

The biological response to stress is a complex, adaptive process involving multiple systems within the body. It's designed to protect an individual by preparing them to react to threats or challenges. However, when this response is constantly activated by the stresses of modern life, it can become harmful. Understanding the biology of stress is crucial for recognizing its impact on health and developing effective strategies to manage it.

The Stress Response System

At the core of the stress response is the hypothalamic-pituitary-adrenal (HPA) axis, a trio of components that play a pivotal role in the body's reaction to stress:

1. Hypothalamus: This brain region initiates the stress response by secreting corticotropin-releasing hormone (CRH).
2. Pituitary Gland: In response to CRH, the pituitary gland releases adrenocorticotropic hormone (ACTH) into the bloodstream.
3. Adrenal Glands: ACTH prompts the adrenal glands, located atop the kidneys, to release cortisol, a primary stress hormone, along with adrenaline (epinephrine) and noradrenaline (norepinephrine).

Cortisol and Its Effects

Cortisol plays a key role in the stress response, helping to mobilize energy by increasing glucose in the bloodstream, enhancing the brain's use of glucose, and increasing the availability of substances that repair tissues. Cortisol also curtails functions that would be nonessential or detrimental in a fight-or-flight situation. It alters immune system responses and suppresses the digestive system, the reproductive system, and growth processes. This complex natural alarm system also communicates with regions of the brain that control mood, motivation, and fear.

Adrenaline and Noradrenaline

Adrenaline and noradrenaline are produced in the adrenal medulla. They are responsible for the immediate physical reactions associated with stress, including increased heart rate, increased blood pressure, and energy surges, preparing the body for rapid action.

The Autonomic Nervous System

The autonomic nervous system, comprising the sympathetic and parasympathetic nervous systems, plays a significant role in the stress response. The sympathetic nervous system triggers the fight-or-flight response, providing the body with a burst of energy to respond to perceived threats. The parasympathetic nervous system helps the body to return to a state of calm once the threat has passed.

Chronic Stress and Health Implications

While the stress response system is self-regulating, with cortisol production inhibiting the HPA axis and restoring equilibrium, chronic stress can disrupt this balance. Prolonged exposure to stress hormones can lead to a host of health problems, including:

- Immune System Suppression: Chronic stress can suppress the immune response, making the body more susceptible to infections and slowing the healing process.

- Cardiovascular Disease: Increased heart rate and blood pressure can raise the risk of hypertension and heart disease.
- Metabolic Syndrome: Chronic stress can contribute to the development of obesity, insulin resistance, and type 2 diabetes.
- Mental Health Issues: Prolonged stress is a significant risk factor for mental health disorders, including anxiety, depression, and PTSD.
- Digestive Problems: Stress can affect the gut, leading to conditions like irritable bowel syndrome (IBS) and gastroesophageal reflux disease (GERD).

Managing the Biological Impact of Stress

Understanding the biology of stress underscores the importance of developing effective stress management techniques. Lifestyle changes, mindfulness practices, physical activity, and seeking professional help can all play a role in mitigating the harmful effects of chronic stress on the body. By addressing stress proactively, individuals can protect their health, improve their quality of life, and enhance their resilience against the inevitable challenges of life.

Stress Reduction Techniques

In the face of the numerous health risks posed by chronic stress, adopting effective stress reduction techniques is essential. These strategies can help mitigate the biological and psychological impacts of stress, promoting overall well-being and resilience. Here are some proven techniques for reducing stress:

1. Mindfulness Meditation

Mindfulness meditation involves paying attention to the present moment without judgment. Regular practice can help reduce stress and anxiety, improve attention, and enhance emotional regulation by fostering a greater awareness of thoughts, feelings, and bodily sensations.

2. Deep Breathing Exercises

Deep breathing techniques, such as diaphragmatic breathing or the 4-7-8 method, can activate the body's relaxation response, counteracting the stress-induced fight-or-flight response. By focusing on slow, deep breaths, these exercises can reduce heart rate and blood pressure, promoting relaxation.

3. Progressive Muscle Relaxation (PMR)

PMR involves tensing and then relaxing each muscle group in the body, promoting physical and mental relaxation. This technique can be particularly effective for reducing stress and tension, as well as improving sleep quality.

4. Physical Activity

Engaging in regular physical activity is one of the most effective stress reduction strategies. Exercise releases endorphins, the body's natural mood lifters, and can also serve as a distraction, allowing individuals to find a quiet moment to break out of the cycle of negative thoughts that feed stress.

5. Yoga and Tai Chi

Yoga and Tai Chi combine physical movement, meditation, and controlled breathing, offering a holistic approach to stress reduction. These practices can help improve flexibility, balance, and strength while also promoting mental calmness and focus.

6. Time in Nature

Spending time in nature, whether it's a walk in the park, gardening, or hiking in the wilderness, can significantly reduce stress levels. Natural settings have been shown to lower cortisol levels, reduce blood pressure, and enhance feelings of well-being.

7. Adequate Sleep

Getting enough sleep is crucial for managing stress. Sleep deprivation can exacerbate stress by impairing cognitive function and emotional regulation. Establishing a regular sleep schedule and creating a calming bedtime routine can improve sleep quality.

8. Social Support

Building and maintaining strong social connections can provide emotional support and reduce the impact of stress. Talking with friends, family, or support groups can offer comfort, advice, and a different perspective on stressful situations.

9. Time Management

Effective time management can alleviate stress caused by feeling overwhelmed. Prioritizing tasks, setting realistic goals, and breaking projects into manageable steps can help reduce the pressure and anxiety associated with a heavy workload.

10. Cognitive-Behavioral Therapy (CBT)

CBT is a type of psychotherapy that can help individuals manage stress by changing negative patterns of thought and behavior. Through CBT, individuals can learn to identify and challenge stressful thoughts, develop coping strategies, and adopt more positive attitudes.

11. Hobbies and Creative Activities

Engaging in hobbies or creative activities can provide a distraction from stress, offering a sense of achievement and joy. Activities like painting, writing, cooking, or playing a musical instrument can serve as effective outlets for stress relief.

Conclusion

Incorporating one or more of these stress reduction techniques into daily life can significantly improve one's ability to manage stress. By actively taking steps to reduce stress, individuals can enhance their health, well-being, and quality of life, building resilience against the challenges that lie ahead.

Positive Psychology and Healing

Positive psychology, a branch of psychology focused on the study of happiness, well-being, and what makes life worth living, offers valuable insights into the healing process. It shifts the focus from pathology and what goes wrong in life to strengths, virtues, and factors that contribute to a high quality of life. This perspective is particularly relevant in the context of healing, as it emphasizes the role of positive emotions, resilience, and optimism in promoting health and well-being.

The Role of Positive Emotions

Research in positive psychology has demonstrated that positive emotions can buffer against stress and contribute to quicker recovery from illness. Emotions such as joy, gratitude, and love not only improve psychological well-being but also have tangible health benefits, including lower blood pressure, reduced risk of heart disease, and improved immune function. Positive emotions can broaden individuals' thought-action repertoires, enabling them to build lasting personal resources and foster resilience.

Resilience and Recovery

Resilience, the ability to bounce back from adversity, plays a crucial role in healing and recovery. Positive psychology explores how resilience can be developed and strengthened through positive emotions, supportive social relationships, and adaptive coping strategies. Resilient individuals are more likely to view challenges as opportunities for growth, maintain a hopeful outlook, and engage in proactive problem-solving, all of which can contribute to more effective healing.

Optimism and Health Outcomes

Optimism, the expectation that good things will happen in the future, has been linked to better health outcomes and longer life expectancy. Optimistic individuals are more likely to engage in healthy behaviors, seek out social support, and adhere to treatment recommendations. They also tend to have lower stress levels and better coping mechanisms, which can positively affect the healing process.

Mindfulness and Present-Moment Awareness

Mindfulness, a key concept in positive psychology, involves paying attention to the present moment with openness, curiosity, and acceptance. Mindfulness practices can reduce stress, anxiety, and depressive symptoms, promoting a sense of calm and well-being. By fostering present-moment awareness, individuals can become more attuned to their bodies' needs and signals, supporting the healing process.

Positive Relationships and Social Support

Positive psychology emphasizes the importance of relationships and social support in promoting health and well-being. Strong, supportive relationships can provide emotional comfort, practical assistance, and a sense of belonging, all of which are beneficial during recovery from illness or injury. Social support can also enhance resilience and encourage positive health behaviors.

Character Strengths and Virtues

Identifying and utilizing one's character strengths and virtues, such as courage, kindness, and perseverance, can empower individuals in their healing journey. Leveraging these strengths can enhance self-esteem, foster resilience, and motivate positive action towards recovery.

Interventions Based on Positive Psychology

Interventions rooted in positive psychology, such as gratitude journaling, practicing acts of kindness, and strength-based therapies, have been shown to improve mental health and can contribute to physical healing. These practices encourage individuals to focus on the positive aspects of their lives, cultivate a sense of purpose, and maintain an optimistic outlook, all of which can enhance the body's ability to heal.

Conclusion

Positive psychology offers a rich framework for understanding and promoting healing. By focusing on strengths, resilience, and positive emotions, individuals can not only navigate the challenges of illness and recovery more effectively but also enhance their overall quality of life. Incorporating principles of positive psychology into health care and daily life can provide a holistic approach to healing, emphasizing the powerful role of the mind and spirit in the process of recovery.

Finding Happiness and Health

The pursuit of happiness is a fundamental human goal, and its connection to health has been extensively explored in the field of positive psychology. Happiness is not just a fleeting emotion but a state that can significantly impact physical health and well-being. Understanding how happiness and health are intertwined reveals the importance of cultivating positive emotions and satisfaction in life as part of a holistic approach to health.

The Bi-directional Relationship between Happiness and Health

Research indicates a bi-directional relationship between happiness and health: not only can good health contribute to happiness, but happiness can also lead to better health outcomes. Happier individuals tend to have stronger immune systems, lower blood pressure, and a reduced risk of chronic diseases. They may also have longer lifespans compared to those who are less happy.

Mechanisms Linking Happiness to Health

- Behavioral Factors: Happier people are more likely to engage in health-promoting behaviors such as regular physical activity, healthy eating, and adequate sleep. They are also less likely to engage in harmful behaviors like smoking and excessive alcohol consumption.
- Biological Factors: Happiness can positively affect biological processes. For instance, it has been linked to lower levels of stress hormones, reduced inflammation, and improved heart health. These biological effects can contribute to a reduced risk of chronic diseases and promote longevity.
- Social Factors: Happiness often leads to greater social engagement and stronger social support networks, which are crucial for mental and physical health. Social connections can provide emotional support, reduce stress, and encourage healthy behaviors.

Cultivating Happiness for Better Health

- Practicing Gratitude: Regularly acknowledging and appreciating the good things in life can enhance happiness and well-being. Keeping a gratitude journal or sharing gratitude with others can deepen relationships and foster a positive outlook.
- Engaging in Acts of Kindness: Helping others and performing acts of kindness can boost happiness levels, create positive social interactions, and enhance feelings of connectedness.
- Fostering Positive Relationships: Investing time and effort into building and maintaining positive relationships can provide emotional support, reduce stress, and contribute to a happier, healthier life.
- Finding Purpose and Meaning: Engaging in activities that feel meaningful can increase happiness, improve mental health, and lead to a more fulfilling life. This can include career pursuits, volunteer work, creative endeavors, or spiritual practices.
- Developing Resilience: Building resilience through positive coping strategies, such as viewing challenges as opportunities for growth, can enhance happiness and well-being, particularly during difficult times.
- Pursuing Goals: Setting and working towards personal goals that align with one's values and interests can provide a sense of accomplishment and satisfaction, contributing to happiness and well-being.

Conclusion

Happiness and health are deeply connected, with each influencing the other in significant ways. By incorporating practices that promote happiness into daily life, individuals can enjoy not only improved mental well-being but also better physical health. Cultivating happiness through gratitude, kindness, positive relationships, purposeful activities, resilience, and goal achievement can lead to a more satisfying and healthier life. Recognizing and embracing the link between happiness and health encourages a comprehensive approach to well-being that encompasses the mind, body, and spirit.

Cultivating Resilience

Resilience, the ability to adapt and bounce back from adversity, stress, and trauma, is a crucial component of psychological health and overall well-being. It enables individuals to navigate life's challenges effectively, maintain mental health during difficult times, and even emerge stronger from such experiences. Cultivating resilience is not an innate trait but a skill that can be developed and strengthened over time through intentional practice and mindset shifts.

Understanding the Foundations of Resilience

Resilience is built on a foundation of several key components, including:

- Emotional Regulation: The ability to manage and respond to emotional experiences in a healthy way.
- Positive Relationships: Supportive social connections that provide encouragement, empathy, and assistance.
- Optimism: A general tendency to expect positive outcomes, coupled with the belief that one has control over one's future.
- Problem-Solving Skills: The ability to identify solutions and take action to resolve difficulties.
- Self-Efficacy: Confidence in one's ability to handle life's challenges.

Strategies for Cultivating Resilience

1. Develop a Growth Mindset: Embrace challenges as opportunities for learning and growth. Understanding that skills and abilities can be developed through effort, good strategies, and input from others encourages resilience.

2. Build Emotional Intelligence: Enhance awareness and understanding of your emotions and those of others. Practice strategies for managing intense emotions, such as mindfulness and self-compassion, to navigate stress and adversity more effectively.

3. Foster Connections: Cultivate strong, positive relationships with family, friends, and community members. Social support is a key factor in resilience, providing emotional comfort and practical help in times of need.

4. Practice Optimism: Focus on the positive aspects of situations and expect good things to happen. Optimism doesn't mean ignoring reality but choosing to maintain a hopeful outlook.

5. Set Realistic Goals: Break tasks into achievable steps. Setting and accomplishing goals, even small ones, can build confidence and a sense of mastery, reinforcing resilience.

6. Embrace Change: Flexibility is an essential part of resilience. Being open to change and adapting to new circumstances can make it easier to navigate life's ups and downs.

7. Take Care of Yourself: Prioritize physical health through regular exercise, a balanced diet, and adequate sleep. Self-care practices enhance your ability to cope with stress and recover from adversity.

8. Seek Purpose: Engage in activities that bring meaning and purpose to your life, whether through work, hobbies, volunteering, or creative pursuits. A sense of purpose can motivate and sustain you through difficult times.

9. Learn from Experiences: Reflect on past adversities and the strategies that helped you overcome them. This reflection can provide valuable insights for dealing with future challenges.

10. Seek Professional Help When Needed: Sometimes, building resilience requires the assistance of a mental health professional. Therapy can provide tools, strategies, and support for developing resilience and coping with life's challenges.

Conclusion

Cultivating resilience is a proactive process that involves developing a set of attitudes, behaviors, and social supports that can help you navigate through life's challenges more effectively. By embracing a growth mindset, fostering strong relationships, practicing self-care, and continually learning from experiences, individuals can build the resilience needed to thrive in the face of adversity. Resilience not only facilitates recovery from difficult situations but also contributes to a richer, more fulfilling life.

Chapter 3: The Physiology of Self-Healing

The human body possesses an innate capacity for self-healing, a complex process involving various physiological mechanisms that repair damage, fight disease, and restore health. Understanding the physiology of self-healing not only highlights the body's remarkable resilience but also underscores the importance of supporting these natural processes through lifestyle choices, stress management, and emotional well-being.

The Immune System and Healing

The immune system is a complex network of cells, tissues, and organs that work in concert to protect the body from infections, diseases, and other potentially harmful foreign bodies. Its role in healing and maintaining health is critical, as it not only fights off pathogens but also plays a part in repairing tissue damage and regulating the body's internal environment. Understanding the immune system's function in healing illuminates the dynamic interplay between defense mechanisms and the body's natural repair processes.

Key Components of the Immune System

- White Blood Cells (Leukocytes): Serve as the frontline defense against pathogens. They are divided into different types, including lymphocytes (B cells and T cells) that target specific pathogens, and phagocytes, which engulf and destroy invaders.
- Antibodies: Proteins produced by B cells that recognize and neutralize foreign invaders such as bacteria and viruses.
- The Complement System: A series of proteins that work in conjunction with antibodies to destroy pathogens.
- The Lymphatic System: Includes lymph nodes, lymph vessels, and lymphocytes, facilitating the transport of immune cells throughout the body and the removal of toxins.
- Bone Marrow: The primary site of new immune cell production.
- The Spleen: Filters the blood, removing old or damaged blood cells and pathogens.
- The Thymus: Where T cells mature and are prepared for their role in immune response.

The Immune Response and Healing

The immune system's response to injury or infection occurs in stages:

1. Innate Immunity: The body's immediate response to injury or infection, involving barriers like the skin and mucous membranes, and nonspecific responses such as inflammation and the activity of phagocytes.
2. Adaptive Immunity: A more targeted response, where the body creates antibodies and activates specific lymphocytes to fight off identified pathogens. This response is slower but more precise, and it provides long-term immunity against future attacks by the same pathogen.

Inflammation as a Healing Response

Inflammation is a vital part of the healing process. When tissues are damaged, the body initiates an inflammatory response to isolate the affected area, remove damaged cells, and fight any infection. Symptoms of inflammation, such as redness, heat, swelling, and pain, signify that healing is underway. Although chronic inflammation can contribute to various diseases, acute inflammation is essential for tissue repair and recovery.

Supporting the Immune System for Optimal Healing

Enhancing the immune system's function can significantly impact the body's ability to heal:

- Nutrition: A diet rich in vitamins, minerals, and antioxidants can bolster the immune response. Key nutrients include vitamin C, vitamin D, zinc, and omega-3 fatty acids.
- Exercise: Regular, moderate exercise has been shown to improve immune function and reduce inflammation.
- Sleep: Adequate sleep is crucial for immune health, as many immune processes are heightened during sleep.
- Stress Management: Chronic stress can suppress immune function. Techniques such as meditation, yoga, and mindfulness can help manage stress levels.
- Hydration: Staying hydrated helps the body produce lymph, a fluid that carries white blood cells and other immune system cells.

Conclusion

The immune system plays a central role in healing, from fighting infections to repairing tissue damage. By understanding its functions and the factors that influence its performance, individuals can take proactive steps to support their immune health. This support not only aids in recovery from injuries and illnesses but also contributes to overall well-being and disease prevention, highlighting the importance of a holistic approach to health that encompasses physical, nutritional, and emotional aspects.

How the Immune System works

The immune system is an intricate and sophisticated defense mechanism that protects the body against infections, diseases, and foreign invaders. It comprises various cells, tissues, and organs that work collaboratively to identify, attack, and eliminate pathogens such as bacteria, viruses, fungi, and parasites. Understanding how the immune system works is essential for grasping its role in maintaining health and facilitating healing.

Components of the Immune System

The immune system can be broadly divided into two main parts: the innate immune system and the adaptive immune system. These two arms work together to provide a comprehensive defense strategy.

Innate Immune System

The innate immune system is the body's first line of defense and responds to pathogens in a generic way. This system acts quickly, often within minutes to hours of an infection:

- Physical Barriers: Skin and mucous membranes act as physical barriers to prevent pathogens from entering the body.
- Chemical Barriers: Substances like stomach acid, enzymes in saliva, and antimicrobial proteins in skin and mucous secretions help destroy invaders.
- Cellular Defenses: Various cells play roles in the innate response, including:
  - Phagocytes: Cells that engulf and digest pathogens. Neutrophils and macrophages are primary phagocytes.
  - Natural Killer (NK) Cells: Lymphocytes that can kill virus-infected cells and tumor cells without prior sensitization to them.
- Inflammatory Response: Triggered by infection or injury, inflammation attracts immune cells to the affected area to eliminate pathogens and begin the healing process.

Adaptive (Acquired) Immune System

The adaptive immune system is more specialized and provides a targeted response to specific pathogens. This system has a memory, allowing for a faster and stronger response upon re-exposure to the same pathogen:

- Lymphocytes: B cells and T cells are the main types of lymphocytes in the adaptive immune system.
  - B Cells: Produce antibodies that bind to antigens (specific proteins on pathogens) to neutralize them or mark them for destruction by other immune cells.
  - T Cells: Include helper T cells, which assist other immune cells; cytotoxic T cells, which kill infected or cancerous cells; and regulatory T cells, which help modulate the immune response.

How the Immune System Works

1. Recognition: The immune system identifies foreign invaders through their antigens. Innate immune cells recognize common features of pathogens, while adaptive immune cells recognize specific antigens.

2. Response: Once a pathogen is identified, the immune system mobilizes its cells to attack and neutralize the threat. The innate response occurs first, followed by the adaptive response if needed.

3. Elimination: Immune cells, such as phagocytes and cytotoxic T cells, work to eliminate the pathogen from the body. B cells produce antibodies that neutralize pathogens or tag them for destruction.

4. Memory: After an infection, the adaptive immune system creates memory cells that remember the specific antigens. If the same pathogen invades again, these memory cells enable the body to respond more quickly and effectively.

Immune System Regulation

To prevent damage to the body's own tissues, the immune system must be tightly regulated. Regulatory mechanisms include the suppression of immune responses once a pathogen is cleared and the prevention of attacks on the body's own cells (autoimmunity).

Conclusion

The immune system's ability to defend against a vast array of pathogens is crucial for survival. Its components work in harmony to detect, respond to, and remember invaders, showcasing the body's remarkable capacity for protection and healing. Understanding the immune system's workings not only highlights the complexity of biological defense mechanisms but also underscores the importance of maintaining immune health through lifestyle choices and, when necessary, medical interventions.

Boosting Immune Function Naturally

Supporting and enhancing the body's immune system through natural means is an integral part of maintaining health and preventing illness. While no single activity or supplement can guarantee immunity from diseases, a combination of healthy lifestyle choices can significantly strengthen the body's natural defense mechanisms. Here are key strategies to naturally boost immune function:

1. Balanced Nutrition

Eating a diet rich in fruits, vegetables, whole grains, lean proteins, and healthy fats can provide essential nutrients that support immune health, including:

- Vitamins A, C, D, and E: Play roles in immune function and can be found in a wide variety of foods like citrus fruits, dark leafy greens, nuts, seeds, and fatty fish.
- Zinc, Selenium, and Iron: Minerals that are critical for immune responses, available in meats, seafood, nuts, and seeds.
- Probiotics: Found in fermented foods like yogurt, kefir, and sauerkraut, probiotics support gut health, which is closely linked to immune function.

2. Regular Physical Activity

Moderate exercise can boost the immune system by promoting good circulation, which allows immune cells and substances to move through the body more effectively. Activities such as walking, cycling, and swimming are beneficial when performed regularly.

3. Adequate Sleep

Sleep and immunity are closely tied. Lack of sleep can impair immune function, so ensuring adequate and quality sleep is vital. Adults should aim for 7-9 hours per night, while children and teenagers need more.

4. Stress Management

Chronic stress can suppress immune function. Techniques such as meditation, deep breathing exercises, yoga, and mindfulness can help manage stress levels, thereby supporting the immune system.

5. Hydration

Staying hydrated helps the body naturally eliminate toxins and other bacteria that may cause illness. Water is best, but herbal teas and other non-caffeinated beverages also contribute to hydration.

6. Healthy Lifestyle Choices

Avoiding smoking, limiting alcohol consumption, and maintaining a healthy weight can further support immune health. These lifestyle choices help reduce the burden on the immune system, allowing it to better fight off infections.

7. Natural Supplements

Certain supplements and herbs are believed to support immune function, including echinacea, elderberry, and garlic. However, it's important to consult with a healthcare provider before starting any supplements, especially for individuals with existing health conditions or those taking medication.

8. Sunlight Exposure

Moderate exposure to sunlight can boost vitamin D levels, which is important for immune function. About 10-15 minutes of sunlight exposure several times a week can help maintain adequate vitamin D levels, but this can vary based on geographic location, skin tone, and time of year.

Conclusion

Boosting immune function naturally involves a holistic approach to health and well-being. By adopting a combination of healthy dietary habits, regular physical activity, adequate sleep, stress management, and other healthy lifestyle choices, individuals can support their immune system and enhance its ability to fight off infections and diseases. It's also crucial to remember that these strategies are part of an overall healthy lifestyle and should complement, not replace, medical advice and treatments when necessary.

Neuroplasticity and Pain Management

Understanding Neuroplasticity

Neuroplasticity, or brain plasticity, refers to the brain's ability to reorganize itself by forming new neural connections throughout life. This adaptability allows the brain to compensate for injury, disease, and adjust to new learning experiences or environmental changes. Neuroplasticity is foundational to understanding how we learn, remember, and recover from brain injuries, but it also plays a significant role in pain management.

The Role of Neuroplasticity in Pain

Pain, especially chronic pain, is not merely a symptom of injury or disease but often involves significant changes in the brain's wiring and function. Neuroplasticity can lead to an increased sensitivity to pain signals (central sensitization), where the brain becomes more efficient at perceiving pain, even in the absence of an actual threat or injury. While this heightened sensitivity is a testament to the brain's adaptability, it can also result in persistent pain that is disproportionate to the physical condition.

Harnessing Neuroplasticity for Pain Management

Understanding neuroplasticity's role in pain offers innovative approaches to pain management. By leveraging the brain's ability to rewire itself, it's possible to develop strategies that reduce pain perception and improve quality of life for those suffering from chronic pain. These strategies include:

- Cognitive Behavioral Therapy (CBT): CBT can help modify the patterns of thinking and behavior related to pain, potentially rewiring the brain's response to pain signals.
- Mindfulness and Meditation: Regular practice can change brain regions associated with pain perception, attention, and emotion regulation, helping to reduce pain and its impact on life.
- Graded Motor Imagery and Mirror Therapy: These therapies can help retrain the brain for those experiencing phantom limb pain or complex regional pain syndrome by gradually re-establishing the connection between motor commands and sensory feedback.
- Physical Therapy and Exercise: Engaging in targeted physical therapy and exercise can promote neuroplastic changes that decrease pain sensitivity and improve function.
- Neurofeedback and Biofeedback: These techniques involve training individuals to control physiological processes that are usually involuntary. For pain management, they can help patients learn to modulate their brain's activity or other physiological responses associated with pain.

The Importance of a Multifaceted Approach

Effective pain management utilizing neuroplasticity often requires a multifaceted approach, combining physical, psychological, and sometimes pharmacological strategies. Tailoring these approaches to the individual's specific condition, preferences, and lifestyle is crucial for optimizing outcomes.

Conclusion

Neuroplasticity's role in pain underscores the complexity of pain perception and management. By understanding and harnessing the brain's ability to reorganize and adapt, individuals suffering from chronic pain have a hopeful avenue for relief and improvement. This understanding also highlights the potential for developing more effective, personalized pain management strategies that address both the physical and psychological aspects of pain.

Leveraging neuroplasticity to rewire the brain is a powerful approach for enhancing cognitive functions, recovering from neurological injuries, and managing conditions like chronic pain. Here are several evidence-based techniques aimed at harnessing the brain's ability to form new neural connections and pathways:

1. Cognitive Behavioral Therapy (CBT)

CBT is a psychotherapeutic treatment that helps individuals identify and challenge negative thought patterns and behaviors. By changing how one thinks about and responds to various situations, CBT can effectively rewire brain circuits associated with emotional regulation, stress response, and pain perception.

2. Mindfulness and Meditation

Practices such as mindfulness meditation have been shown to produce changes in brain regions related to attention, emotion regulation, and self-awareness. Regular meditation can increase the gray matter density in the prefrontal cortex, hippocampus, and other areas, enhancing cognitive functions and emotional well-being.

3. Physical Exercise

Exercise promotes neurogenesis (the creation of new neurons) and increases synaptic plasticity, improving learning, memory, and cognitive flexibility. Aerobic exercises, in particular, can lead to growth in brain areas such as the hippocampus, which is crucial for memory and learning.

4. Learning New Skills

Engaging in new learning activities stimulates the brain, encouraging the growth of new neural connections. Activities that challenge the brain, such as learning a new language, instrument, or hobby, can enhance cognitive abilities and promote neuroplasticity.

5. Graded Motor Imagery (GMI)

GMI is a therapeutic process used primarily for pain management and neurological rehabilitation. It involves several stages, including left/right discrimination, motor imagery, and mirror therapy, aimed at gradually retraining the brain's perception of movement and pain.

6. Neurofeedback

Neurofeedback trains individuals to control their brain activity by providing real-time feedback on brain wave patterns. This technique can improve attention, reduce anxiety, and alleviate symptoms of various neurological disorders by promoting specific patterns of brain activity.

7. Positive Reinforcement and Reward-Based Learning

Positive reinforcement and reward-based learning can strengthen desired neural pathways. Engaging in activities that bring joy and satisfaction can release dopamine, a neurotransmitter that plays a key role in motivation, pleasure, and learning, thereby reinforcing positive behaviors and thought patterns.

8. Mind-Body Techniques

Other mind-body techniques, such as yoga and tai chi, combine physical movement, breath control, and meditation to improve mental and physical health. These practices can enhance body awareness, reduce stress, and contribute to brain health and neuroplasticity.

9. Dietary Adjustments

A nutrient-rich diet supports brain health and cognitive function. Omega-3 fatty acids, antioxidants, vitamins, and minerals can protect brain cells, reduce inflammation, and support the growth of new neurons.

10. Quality Sleep

Adequate and quality sleep is essential for neuroplasticity. During sleep, the brain consolidates memories, clears out toxins, and repairs itself, supporting learning and memory and facilitating the formation of new neural connections.

Conclusion

Harnessing neuroplasticity through these techniques offers immense potential for improving brain health, cognitive function, and overall well-being. Whether recovering from injury, managing chronic conditions, or simply aiming to enhance cognitive abilities, incorporating these practices into daily life can lead to significant positive changes in brain structure and function.

The Gut-Brain Axis

The gut-brain axis represents the complex communication network that links the enteric nervous system (ENS) of the gastrointestinal tract with the central nervous system (CNS), which includes the brain and spinal cord. This bidirectional communication pathway involves direct and indirect connections facilitated by neural, hormonal, and immunological mechanisms, playing a crucial role in maintaining overall health and influencing a wide range of physiological processes.

The Role of Gut Health

Gut health is pivotal within the context of the gut-brain axis, significantly impacting mental health, immune response, and even the body's ability to manage stress. The gut microbiome, consisting of trillions of microorganisms, including bacteria, viruses, and fungi, is essential in this interplay, affecting everything from nutrient absorption and immune system modulation to neurotransmitter production.

Impact on Mental Health

The gut microbiome can influence brain chemistry and behavior, contributing to the development or mitigation of various mental health disorders, including anxiety, depression, and autism spectrum disorders. Microbes in the gut produce neurotransmitters like serotonin and gamma-aminobutyric acid (GABA), which play roles in mood regulation. Dysbiosis, or an imbalance in the gut microbiota, has been linked to changes in mood and cognitive functions, underscoring the importance of gut health in mental well-being.

Immune System Modulation

The gut is a key immune organ, with a substantial portion of the body's immune cells residing in the gut-associated lymphoid tissue (GALT). The microbiome plays a critical role in training and regulating the immune system, distinguishing between harmless substances and potential pathogens. A healthy gut microbiome can prevent the development of autoimmune diseases and allergies by promoting immune tolerance and reducing inflammation.

Stress Response

The gut-brain axis also influences the body's response to stress. Stress can affect gut permeability, leading to a condition colloquially known as "leaky gut," which can trigger or exacerbate inflammation and immune responses. Conversely, a healthy gut can contribute to a more resilient stress response, potentially mitigating the negative impacts of chronic stress on the body.

Strategies to Support Gut Health

- Diet: Consuming a diverse diet rich in whole foods, fibers, and fermented products can support a healthy microbiome. Prebiotic and probiotic foods encourage the growth of beneficial bacteria.
- Avoid Overuse of Antibiotics: While sometimes necessary, antibiotics can disrupt the gut microbiota. Use them judiciously and always under medical guidance.
- Manage Stress: Chronic stress can negatively affect gut health. Engaging in stress-reduction practices like meditation, exercise, and adequate sleep can help maintain a healthy gut.
- Regular Exercise: Physical activity can enhance the diversity and health of the gut microbiome, contributing to improved gut and overall health.

Conclusion

The gut-brain axis is a fundamental aspect of human physiology, illustrating the profound interconnectedness of mental and physical health. By understanding and nurturing gut health through diet, lifestyle choices, and stress management, individuals can positively influence their mental well-being, immune function, and resilience to stress, highlighting the importance of a holistic approach to health that considers the intricate relationships within the body.

Diet and Mental Well-being

The connection between diet and mental well-being is a critical component of overall health, emphasizing the significant impact of nutrition on cognitive function, mood, and emotional health. Scientific research increasingly supports the notion that what we eat not only affects our physical health but also has profound implications for our mental state.

Nutritional Psychiatry

Nutritional psychiatry is an emerging field focused on the role of nutrition in the development, prevention, and treatment of mental health disorders. It investigates how dietary patterns and specific nutrients contribute to brain health and explores dietary interventions as potential strategies for improving mental well-being.

Key Nutrients for Mental Health

- Omega-3 Fatty Acids: Found in fatty fish (such as salmon, mackerel, and sardines), flaxseeds, and walnuts, omega-3s are essential for brain function and have been linked to reduced rates of depression and anxiety.
- B Vitamins: B vitamins, particularly B12, B6, and folate, play roles in neurotransmitter synthesis and brain function. Deficiencies have been associated with increased risk of depression and mood disturbances. Sources include leafy greens, legumes, meats, and fortified foods.
- Antioxidants: Vitamins C and E, selenium, and flavonoids can combat oxidative stress in the brain, which is linked to mood disorders. Berries, nuts, seeds, and vegetables are rich in antioxidants.
- Probiotics and Prebiotics: Supporting gut health through the consumption of probiotic (yogurt, kefir, sauerkraut) and prebiotic foods (garlic, onions, bananas) can positively impact mental health via the gut-brain axis.

The Impact of Diet Patterns on Mental Health

- Mediterranean Diet: Characterized by a high intake of vegetables, fruits, nuts, seeds, legumes, whole grains, fish, and olive oil, the Mediterranean diet has been associated with a lower risk of depression and cognitive decline.
- Western Diet: High consumption of processed foods, red meat, high-fat dairy products, and sugary snacks has been linked to an increased risk of depression, anxiety, and other mental health disorders.

Dietary Interventions for Mental Health

Implementing dietary changes as part of a comprehensive approach to mental health can offer several benefits:

- Improved Mood: A nutritious diet can enhance mood by regulating blood sugar levels and providing essential nutrients that support neurotransmitter function.
- Reduced Anxiety and Stress: Certain dietary patterns and nutrients can modulate the body's stress response and support resilience against anxiety.
- Cognitive Function: Adequate nutrition supports brain health and cognitive function, potentially reducing the risk of age-related cognitive decline and dementia.

Practical Tips for a Mental Health-Friendly Diet

- Prioritize Whole Foods: Focus on consuming a variety of whole foods that provide a broad spectrum of nutrients.
- Limit Processed Foods and Sugar: Reducing intake of processed foods and added sugars can help stabilize mood and energy levels.
- Stay Hydrated: Adequate hydration is important for cognitive function and overall well-being.
- Mindful Eating: Pay attention to how food affects your mood and energy levels, adjusting your diet accordingly.

Conclusion

The relationship between diet and mental well-being is complex and multifaceted, encompassing the direct effects of nutrients on brain chemistry and the broader impact of dietary patterns on overall health. By recognizing the importance of nutrition in mental health, individuals can make informed choices that support both their physical and mental well-being, contributing to a holistic approach to health that acknowledges the intricate connection between the mind and body.

Chapter 4: Mindfulness and Meditation

The Basics of Mindfulness

Mindfulness is a practice rooted in ancient meditation traditions, now widely embraced in various forms across the world for its benefits to mental and physical health. At its core, mindfulness involves paying attention to the present moment with an attitude of openness, curiosity, and non-judgment. It encourages an awareness of one's thoughts, emotions, bodily sensations, and surrounding environment without clinging to them or pushing them away.

Key Components of Mindfulness:

- Attention: The practice of directing one's focus to the present experience, observing thoughts, feelings, and sensations as they arise.
- Acceptance: Approaching each moment with acceptance, rather than judgment or avoidance, acknowledging experiences without trying to change them.
- Awareness: Cultivating a heightened state of awareness that allows for greater insight into the nature of one's mind and the external world.

Mindfulness in Daily Life

Incorporating mindfulness into daily life doesn't necessarily require setting aside large blocks of time for meditation. While formal meditation practices are beneficial, mindfulness can also be practiced in everyday activities by adopting a mindful attitude towards one's experiences. Here are ways to integrate mindfulness into daily routines:

Mindful Eating:

- Engage fully with the experience of eating, paying attention to the taste, texture, and aroma of food. Notice the colors on your plate and the sensations of hunger and fullness, eating slowly and without distraction.

Mindful Walking:

- Turn routine walks into mindfulness exercises by focusing on the sensation of movement and the contact of your feet with the ground. Observe the sights, sounds, and smells around you, bringing your attention back to the present whenever it wanders.

Mindful Listening:

- Practice active, attentive listening in conversations, fully focusing on the speaker without formulating responses in your mind or becoming distracted by external factors.

Mindful Breathing:

- Take short breaks throughout the day to focus on your breath. Notice the sensation of air entering and leaving your nostrils and the rise and fall of your chest, using the breath as an anchor to the present moment.

Mindful Observation:

- Choose an object from your environment and observe it with fresh eyes, as if seeing it for the first time. Notice its colors, textures, and features, appreciating its presence without attaching labels or judgments.

Benefits of Mindfulness in Daily Life

Practicing mindfulness in everyday activities can offer numerous benefits, including:

- Reduced Stress: By focusing on the present, mindfulness helps reduce rumination and worry about the past or future, lowering stress levels.
- Enhanced Emotional Regulation: Mindfulness fosters an awareness of emotional responses, allowing for more thoughtful reactions and reducing impulsivity.
- Improved Concentration: Regular mindfulness practice can enhance focus and attention, making it easier to engage fully in tasks.
- Increased Enjoyment: Being present in the moment can enhance the enjoyment of daily activities, leading to greater satisfaction and well-being.
- Better Physical Health: Mindfulness has been linked to lower blood pressure, improved sleep, and a stronger immune system.

Conclusion

Mindfulness offers a simple yet profound way to engage with our lives, promoting greater awareness, acceptance, and appreciation of the present moment. By weaving mindfulness into daily activities, individuals can cultivate a more peaceful, balanced, and fulfilling life, enhancing both mental and physical health.

Mindful Awareness Practices

Mindful awareness practices (MAPs) are structured techniques designed to cultivate mindfulness, the quality of being fully present and engaged in the moment, aware of your thoughts and feelings without distraction or judgment. These practices are foundational to developing a deeper sense of awareness and connection to the present moment, enhancing overall well-being and reducing stress. Here's an overview of several key MAPs and how they can be integrated into daily life.

1. Sitting Meditation

Sitting meditation is a cornerstone of mindful awareness practices. It involves sitting in a comfortable, upright position, focusing on the breath or a mantra, and observing thoughts and sensations without attachment as they arise and pass.

- How to Practice: Choose a quiet spot. Sit on a chair or cushion with your back straight. Close your eyes or lower your gaze. Focus on your breath, noticing the sensation of air moving in and out of your nostrils, or the rise and fall of your chest. When your mind wanders, gently bring your attention back to your breath.

2. Body Scan Meditation

Body scan meditation promotes awareness and relaxation by directing attention to different parts of the body, noting sensations without judgment.

- How to Practice: Lie down or sit comfortably. Close your eyes and take a few deep breaths. Starting at your feet, gradually move your attention up through your body, noticing sensations, tension, or warmth in each area. Breathe into any areas of tension, imagining them relaxing with each exhale.

3. Mindful Walking

Mindful walking combines movement with mindfulness, encouraging awareness of the physical experience of walking, the environment, and the sensations in the body.

- How to Practice: Walk at a relaxed, slow pace. Focus on the sensation of your feet touching the ground, the rhythm of your steps, and the movement of your body. Observe the sights, sounds, and smells around you, bringing your attention back to the act of walking whenever your mind wanders.

4. Mindful Eating

Mindful eating involves paying full attention to the experience of eating, appreciating the flavors, textures, and sensations, and listening to the body's hunger and fullness cues.

- How to Practice: Begin by observing your food, noticing its colors and aromas. Chew slowly, savoring each bite and paying attention to the taste and texture. Be aware of your body's hunger and fullness signals, eating until you are satisfied but not overly full.

5. Loving-kindness Meditation (Metta)

Loving-kindness meditation fosters an attitude of compassion and kindness towards oneself and others. It involves silently repeating phrases of goodwill and kindness, directing them towards oneself, loved ones, acquaintances, and even those with whom one has difficulties.

- How to Practice: Sit comfortably and close your eyes. Begin by directing kind phrases towards yourself, such as "May I be happy, may I be healthy, may I be at peace." Gradually extend these wishes to others, visualizing each person and offering them your goodwill.

Benefits of Mindful Awareness Practices

Practicing MAPs regularly can offer numerous psychological and physiological benefits, including:

- Reduced Stress and Anxiety: By focusing on the present, MAPs help break the cycle of rumination and worry.
- Improved Mood and Emotional Regulation: Regular practice can enhance mood and provide tools for managing emotional responses more effectively.
- Enhanced Focus and Concentration: Mindfulness practices can improve the ability to maintain attention and concentrate on tasks.
- Greater Physical Well-being: MAPs have been associated with lower blood pressure, improved sleep quality, and a stronger immune system.

Conclusion

Mindful awareness practices offer accessible, flexible tools for enhancing mindfulness in everyday life. By incorporating these practices into your routine, you can cultivate a deeper sense of presence, awareness, and compassion, leading to improved mental, emotional, and physical well-being. Whether through sitting meditation, mindful walking, or loving-kindness meditation, the journey towards mindfulness begins with a single, intentional moment of awareness.

Meditation Techniques for Healing

Meditation has been used for centuries as a method for achieving mental clarity, emotional calm, and physical relaxation. Today, it is widely recognized for its healing properties, offering relief from stress, anxiety, chronic pain, and a variety of health conditions. Understanding the different types of meditation can help individuals find the most suitable practice for their healing journey.

Types of Meditation

1. Mindfulness Meditation

Mindfulness meditation originates from Buddhist teachings and is one of the most popular meditation techniques in the West. It involves paying attention to the present moment, observing thoughts, feelings, and bodily sensations without judgment.

- Healing Benefits: Reduces stress, improves mental health, enhances emotional regulation, and can alleviate symptoms of anxiety and depression.

2. Transcendental Meditation (TM)

Transcendental Meditation is a simple, natural technique practiced for 20 minutes twice a day while sitting comfortably with the eyes closed. It involves silently repeating a mantra to facilitate a unique state of restful alertness.

- Healing Benefits: Lowers blood pressure, reduces stress and anxiety, and improves heart health.

3. Guided Meditation

Also known as guided imagery or visualization, this technique involves forming mental images of places or situations you find relaxing. It's often led by a guide or teacher, making it an accessible form of meditation for beginners.

- Healing Benefits: Promotes relaxation, reduces stress, and can help manage pain by directing attention away from discomfort.

4. Loving-kindness Meditation (Metta)

Loving-kindness meditation focuses on developing feelings of goodwill, kindness, and warmth towards oneself and others. Practitioners repeat positive phrases or wishes for themselves and extend them to others, including friends, acquaintances, and even those with whom they have conflict.

- Healing Benefits: Increases positive emotions, reduces negative emotions like anxiety and depression, and enhances feelings of social connectedness.

5. Body Scan Meditation

This form of meditation encourages individuals to scan their body for areas of tension, noting any sensations or discomfort without trying to change them. It's often used in mindfulness-based stress reduction (MBSR) programs.

- Healing Benefits: Helps with stress and pain management, improves body awareness, and can lead to greater emotional calm.

6. Zen Meditation (Zazen)

Zen meditation, or Zazen, is a form of seated meditation that is a foundational practice in Zen Buddhism. Practitioners sit in a specific posture and focus on their breath, sometimes concentrating on the movement of air through the nose or the rise and fall of the abdomen.

- Healing Benefits: Enhances focus and concentration, reduces stress, and fosters a sense of peace and self-awareness.

7. Yoga Meditation

Yoga incorporates physical postures (asanas), breath control (pranayama), and meditation. It is a holistic practice that unites the body, mind, and spirit, offering a variety of meditation styles within its practice.

- Healing Benefits: Improves physical flexibility and strength, reduces stress, and supports mental clarity and inner peace.

Conclusion

Meditation offers a versatile array of techniques suitable for addressing a wide range of physical, mental, and emotional health issues. By exploring different types of meditation, individuals can discover the practices that resonate most with their healing needs, cultivating a sense of balance, well-being, and inner peace. Whether seeking relief from stress, pain, or seeking deeper self-awareness, meditation provides accessible tools for nurturing health and promoting healing.

Establishing a Meditation Practice

Creating a consistent meditation practice is a transformative process that can significantly improve your quality of life, offering benefits for your mental, emotional, and physical health. However, establishing a routine can be challenging at first. Here are practical steps and tips to help you create and maintain a regular meditation practice.

1. Start Small

Begin with short meditation sessions, even just a few minutes a day. Gradually increase the duration as you become more comfortable with the practice. Starting small helps prevent overwhelm and makes the habit more manageable and sustainable.

2. Set a Regular Time

Choose a specific time of day for your meditation practice. Many people find that meditating first thing in the morning or right before bed works well for them. Consistency in timing helps establish meditation as a daily habit.

3. Create a Dedicated Space

Designate a quiet, comfortable spot in your home where you can meditate without interruptions. Having a dedicated space can enhance your practice and make it easier to enter a meditative state. Consider adding elements that promote relaxation, such as cushions, a mat, or calming decorations.

4. Use Guided Meditations

If you're new to meditation or find it challenging to focus, guided meditations can be extremely helpful. Many apps, websites, and videos offer guided sessions for various meditation styles and durations. Guided practices provide structure and can teach you fundamental techniques.

5. Explore Different Techniques

There are many types of meditation (e.g., mindfulness, loving-kindness, body scan, etc.). Experiment with different methods to find what resonates with you. Variety can keep your practice interesting and address different aspects of your well-being.

6. Make It a Priority

Treat your meditation practice as an important appointment with yourself. Schedule it into your day and commit to it as you would any other essential activity. Remind yourself of the benefits to stay motivated.

7. Be Patient and Kind to Yourself

Meditation is a skill that takes time to develop. You might encounter distractions, boredom, or resistance along the way. Practice self-compassion and patience. Each session is an opportunity to learn and grow, regardless of its perceived success.

8. Keep a Meditation Journal

Recording your experiences, thoughts, and feelings after each meditation session can deepen your practice. A journal allows you to reflect on your progress, notice patterns, and gain insights into your mental and emotional states.

9. Join a Meditation Group

Participating in a meditation group or community can provide support, motivation, and deeper learning. Sharing your practice with others offers accountability and can enhance your commitment.

10. Incorporate Mindfulness into Daily Activities

Extend mindfulness beyond your meditation sessions by practicing it during everyday activities. Pay attention to your breath, sensations, and surroundings while eating, walking, or engaging in other routine tasks. This continuous practice can significantly enrich your experience.

Conclusion

Establishing a meditation practice is a journey of personal exploration and growth. By starting small, creating a conducive environment, and being patient with yourself, you can develop a meaningful practice that enhances your well-being. Remember, the key to successful meditation is consistency, not perfection. With time and dedication, meditation can become a valuable and rewarding part of your daily routine.

The Science Behind Mindfulness and Meditation

The increasing interest in mindfulness and meditation over recent years is backed by a growing body of scientific research. These practices, once considered purely spiritual or relaxation techniques, are now recognized for their tangible physiological benefits. Understanding the science behind mindfulness and meditation reveals how these practices can significantly impact health and well-being.

Physiological Benefits

1. Stress Reduction

One of the most well-documented benefits of mindfulness and meditation is stress reduction. Practices like mindfulness-based stress reduction (MBSR) have been shown to lower cortisol levels, the body's primary stress hormone. This reduction in cortisol can alleviate the physical and psychological effects of stress, including inflammation and high blood pressure.

2. Improved Immune Function

Regular meditation has been linked to improved immune function. Studies suggest that mindfulness practices can increase the activity of natural killer cells, which are crucial for the body's defense against viruses and cancerous cells. Meditation may also influence genes related to immunity, enhancing the body's resistance to illness.

3. Enhanced Brain Function

Mindfulness and meditation can lead to structural changes in the brain, a phenomenon known as neuroplasticity. Research using MRI scans has shown increased gray matter density in areas of the brain associated with memory, learning, and emotion regulation, such as the hippocampus and prefrontal cortex. Additionally, meditation can decrease the size of the amygdala, the brain region involved in stress and fear responses.

4. Better Cardiovascular Health

Meditation practices can positively affect heart health by reducing risk factors for cardiovascular disease. Benefits include lower blood pressure, reduced heart rate, decreased inflammation, and improved blood circulation. These changes can lower the risk of heart disease and stroke.

5. Pain Management

Meditation can alter the perception of pain in the brain. By fostering a non-judgmental awareness of pain sensations, mindfulness can reduce the emotional response to pain and decrease overall discomfort. Studies have shown that meditation can be an effective complement to traditional pain management strategies.

6. Enhanced Emotional Well-being

Practicing mindfulness and meditation promotes emotional stability and psychological well-being. These practices can reduce symptoms of anxiety, depression, and emotional distress by improving emotional regulation and reducing rumination.

7. Improved Sleep

Mindfulness meditation can improve the quality of sleep by helping to quiet the mind and reduce stress levels, making it easier to fall asleep and stay asleep. Meditation practices have been used successfully as a treatment for insomnia and other sleep disorders.

Conclusion

The science behind mindfulness and meditation offers compelling evidence of their benefits for physical and mental health. Through various physiological changes — from reduced stress levels and enhanced immune function to improved brain function and cardiovascular health — mindfulness and meditation practices can play a significant role in promoting overall well-being. As research continues to evolve, it underscores the potential of these practices as powerful tools for enhancing health and quality of life.

Psychological Effects of Mindfulness and Meditation

Mindfulness and meditation not only offer substantial physiological benefits but also have a profound impact on psychological well-being. These practices have been extensively studied for their ability to improve mental health, enhance cognitive functions, and contribute to emotional stability. Here's an overview of the key psychological effects of mindfulness and meditation.

1. Reduced Symptoms of Anxiety and Depression

Mindfulness meditation has been shown to significantly reduce symptoms of anxiety and depression. By promoting an attitude of acceptance and non-judgment, it helps individuals break free from patterns of negative thinking and rumination that often underlie these conditions. Regular practice can lead to changes in brain areas related to mood regulation, such as increased activity in the prefrontal cortex and reduced activity in the amygdala.

2. Enhanced Emotional Regulation

Practicing mindfulness enhances the ability to regulate emotions by increasing awareness of emotional states and providing strategies to manage them more effectively. This increased emotional intelligence allows for better handling of stress, adversity, and challenging interpersonal dynamics, contributing to more adaptive responses and healthier relationships.

3. Improved Attention and Concentration

One of the foundational elements of mindfulness is the cultivation of focused attention. Studies have shown that regular meditation practice can improve concentration, attention span, and the ability to multitask, with changes observed in brain regions associated with attentional control. These benefits can translate into improved performance in academic, professional, and personal settings.

4. Increased Self-awareness and Insight

Mindfulness practices foster a deeper level of self-awareness and insight by encouraging individuals to observe their thoughts, feelings, and behaviors without judgment. This introspective practice can lead to a better understanding of oneself, including recognizing patterns of thought and behavior that may not serve one's well-being, thereby facilitating personal growth and development.

5. Enhanced Resilience to Stress

By changing the way individuals relate to stress, mindfulness and meditation can enhance resilience. Practitioners learn to view stressors more objectively and respond to challenges with a greater sense of calm and clarity. This shift in perspective can reduce the psychological impact of stress and help individuals bounce back more quickly from difficult situations.

6. Improved Sleep Quality

Mindfulness meditation can improve sleep quality by helping individuals relax and reduce the mental chatter that often interferes with falling asleep. By addressing underlying stress and anxiety, mindfulness can also contribute to a more restful night's sleep, further supporting psychological well-being.

7. Greater Overall Well-being and Life Satisfaction

The cumulative effect of practicing mindfulness and meditation is often an increased sense of overall well-being and life satisfaction. Individuals report feeling more present, connected, and fulfilled in their daily lives, with a greater capacity for joy, gratitude, and compassion towards themselves and others.

Conclusion

The psychological effects of mindfulness and meditation are broad and deeply transformative. These practices offer effective tools for managing mental health, enhancing cognitive abilities, and fostering emotional growth. As mindfulness and meditation continue to gain recognition and acceptance in the field of psychology, they represent vital components of a holistic approach to mental health and well-being, accessible to individuals seeking to enrich their lives and navigate the complexities of the human experience.

Chapter 5: Visualization and Imagery

Principles of Visualization

Visualization, also known as mental imagery or guided imagery, is a powerful technique that involves creating vivid, detailed images in the mind. This practice is rooted in the principle that the mind and body are interconnected, and mental images can influence physical and emotional states. Visualization leverages this mind-body connection to promote healing, improve performance, and achieve specific goals. Understanding the principles behind visualization is key to effectively utilizing this technique.

Key Principles Include:

- Vividness: The more detailed and vivid the mental image, the more effective the visualization. Incorporating all five senses—sight, sound, touch, taste, and smell—can enhance the vividness and impact of the imagery.
- Emotion: Incorporating emotional elements into visualization strengthens its effect. Positive emotions associated with the mental images can enhance motivation and engagement with the goals or outcomes being visualized.
- Repetition: Regular practice of visualization reinforces the desired outcomes or behaviors. Consistency strengthens the neural pathways associated with the visualized scenarios, making them more accessible and influential over time.
- Belief: A strong belief in the possibility of the desired outcome and the effectiveness of visualization is crucial. Confidence in the process can enhance the impact of the imagery on thoughts, feelings, and physiological responses.
- Relaxation: Starting visualization from a state of relaxation can facilitate deeper engagement with the imagery. Relaxation techniques such as deep breathing or progressive muscle relaxation can help prepare the mind and body for effective visualization.

How Visualization Works

Visualization works by engaging the brain's inherent ability to imagine and simulate experiences, affecting both psychological and physiological processes. Despite the absence of actual external stimuli, the brain can respond to vividly imagined scenarios as if they were real, triggering similar neural activations, emotional responses, and even physical reactions.

Mechanisms of Action:

- Neural Activation: Imaging studies have shown that visualization activates many of the same brain areas involved in actual perception and action. For instance, visualizing playing a piano piece can activate similar brain regions as physically playing the instrument.
- Psychoneuroimmunology (PNI): Visualization can influence the immune system through psychological states. Positive imagery can enhance mood and reduce stress, indirectly supporting immune function and promoting healing.
- Autonomic Nervous System (ANS) Response: Visualization can affect the ANS, which controls bodily functions like heart rate and digestion. For example, visualizing a peaceful scene can induce a relaxation response, lowering stress and its physiological effects.

- Placebo Effect: Visualization can harness the placebo effect, where belief in the effectiveness of a non-active treatment leads to real improvements. Imagining positive health outcomes can trigger changes in the body that contribute to healing or improved well-being.
- Performance Enhancement: Athletes, performers, and professionals use visualization to prepare for events, rehearse skills, and enhance confidence. Mentally practicing skills can improve actual performance, likely due to the strengthening of neural pathways associated with the visualized activities.

Conclusion

Visualization and imagery harness the power of the mind to influence both mental and physical health. By understanding and applying the principles of vividness, emotion, repetition, belief, and relaxation, individuals can effectively utilize visualization to support healing, achieve personal goals, and enhance performance. As a testament to the interconnectedness of mind and body, visualization offers a versatile and accessible tool for personal development and well-being.

Creating Effective Visualizations

Effective visualizations are a powerful tool for personal development, healing, and achieving goals. They involve creating vivid, detailed mental images that evoke positive emotions and sensations, influencing both the mind and body. To create impactful visualizations, certain techniques and principles can be applied, enhancing their effectiveness and the likelihood of achieving desired outcomes.

Steps to Creating Effective Visualizations:

1. Define Your Goal Clearly: Start with a clear, specific objective. Whether it's improving health, achieving a performance goal, or enhancing well-being, knowing exactly what you want to achieve sets the foundation for effective visualization (Achterberg, 1985).

2. Enter a Relaxed State: Begin your visualization practice in a state of relaxation. Deep breathing, progressive muscle relaxation, or gentle stretching can help calm the mind and body, making it easier to focus on your imagery (Rossman, 2000).

3. Use All Senses: Make your visualization as vivid and detailed as possible by incorporating all five senses. Imagine not just what you see, but also what you hear, feel, smell, and taste. This multisensory approach engages the brain more fully, enhancing the impact of the visualization (Cumming & Ramsey, 2009).

4. Incorporate Emotion: The emotional component of visualization is crucial. Try to feel the emotions associated with achieving your goal or experiencing your desired outcome. Positive emotions like joy, pride, and gratitude can amplify the effects of visualization (Holmes & Mathews, 2010).

5. Practice Regularly: Like any skill, visualization becomes more effective with practice. Consistent, daily practice reinforces the neural pathways associated with your visualized goals, making them more attainable (Ersdal, 2008).

6. Use First-person Perspective: Visualize from a first-person perspective, seeing the scenario unfold through your own eyes rather than as an observer. This perspective can create a more immersive and personal experience, strengthening the connection to the visualized outcome (Hale, 1994).

7. Incorporate Movement: If applicable, visualize not only the outcome but also the actions leading up to it. For performance goals, imagine performing the actions smoothly and confidently. This technique is particularly beneficial for athletes and performers, reinforcing muscle memory and skill (Driskell, Copper, & Moran, 1994).

8. Utilize Guided Imagery: For those new to visualization or seeking structured practice, guided imagery sessions led by a therapist or through audio recordings can provide a framework for effective visualization. These guided sessions often include detailed scenarios designed to promote relaxation, healing, or goal achievement (Rossman, 2000).

Conclusion

Creating effective visualizations is a dynamic process that benefits from clarity, sensory detail, emotional engagement, and regular practice. By applying these principles, individuals can harness the power of their imagination to foster healing, enhance performance, and achieve personal growth, illustrating the profound impact of the mind on both psychological and physiological well-being.

How Imagery Promotes Healing

The Power of Mental Images

The use of imagery for healing, a practice rooted in ancient traditions and validated by contemporary science, harnesses the power of mental images to influence physical health, emotional well-being, and recovery processes. Understanding how imagery promotes healing involves recognizing the interconnectedness of the mind and body and the significant impact that one's mental state can have on physical health.

The Power of Mental Images

Mental images are more than mere thoughts or daydreams; they are vivid, multisensory experiences created in the mind that can have profound physiological and psychological effects. These images, when harnessed with intention and focus, can stimulate real physical and emotional responses, mirroring those that might occur in response to actual external stimuli.

Mechanisms of Healing Through Imagery

1. Stress Reduction: Imagery can induce relaxation and reduce stress by activating the parasympathetic nervous system, counterbalancing the body's stress response. This relaxation response can lower blood pressure, reduce heart rate, and decrease muscle tension, creating optimal conditions for the body to heal.

2. Enhanced Immune Function: There is evidence to suggest that positive mental imagery can boost immune function. By visualizing the immune system effectively identifying and eliminating pathogens, individuals may be able to enhance their body's natural defense mechanisms against illness and infection.

3. Pain Management: Imagery can alter the perception of pain by changing the way pain signals are processed in the brain. Visualizing oneself in a pain-free state or engaging the mind with positive, absorbing images can distract from pain and reduce its intensity.

4. Improved Self-Efficacy and Motivation: Imagery can bolster self-efficacy—the belief in one's ability to achieve specific goals, including health-related ones. By visualizing successful outcomes, whether it's recovering from surgery, managing chronic illness, or achieving personal wellness goals, individuals can enhance their motivation and resilience, key factors in the healing process.

5. Emotional and Psychological Healing: Imagery can be used to explore and resolve emotional and psychological issues contributing to physical symptoms or conditions. Visualizing safe, healing environments or positive, affirming experiences can help process emotional trauma, reduce anxiety and depression, and promote a sense of peace and well-being.

How to Utilize Healing Imagery

- Guided Imagery: Working with a therapist or using pre-recorded audio guides can provide structured imagery exercises tailored to specific health goals or challenges.

- Personalized Imagery: Creating personal images that evoke a sense of calm, strength, or healing can be particularly powerful. These might include visualizing a peaceful natural setting, imagining the body healing at the cellular level, or seeing oneself achieving a desired health outcome.

- Consistent Practice: Regular practice strengthens the effectiveness of imagery for healing. Setting aside dedicated time each day for imagery exercises can enhance their impact over time.

Conclusion

The power of mental images to promote healing highlights the profound influence of the mind on the body. By engaging in visualization and imagery practices, individuals can tap into their inner resources for stress reduction, pain management, and emotional healing, complementing traditional medical treatments and supporting overall well-being. Whether used for addressing specific health issues or enhancing general wellness, the practice of imagery for healing offers a versatile and accessible tool for harnessing the mind-body connection.

Success Stories: The Impact of Visualization and Imagery on Healing

The practice of visualization and imagery for healing has been embraced across various fields, from sports psychology to medical treatment, due to its profound impact on performance, recovery, and overall well-being. These success stories from individuals and research studies highlight the transformative power of mental imagery in facilitating healing, enhancing abilities, and achieving remarkable outcomes.

Overcoming Physical Injuries

Athletes have long used visualization techniques to recover from injuries. One notable example involves a professional basketball player who sustained a significant knee injury. During his rehabilitation, he not only adhered to his physical therapy regimen but also consistently visualized his knee healing and himself performing at his peak level on the court. This dual approach significantly contributed to his successful return to professional play, with a recovery time that surpassed medical expectations. The mental imagery not only aided his physical recovery but also maintained his confidence and competitive edge.

Enhancing Surgical Recovery

A study involving patients undergoing surgery found that those who participated in guided imagery sessions before and after the operation experienced less pain, reduced anxiety, and faster recovery times compared to those who received standard care alone. Patients used visualization techniques to imagine the surgical process going smoothly, their bodies healing quickly, and themselves recovering strongly. This mind-body intervention demonstrated how positive mental imagery could significantly impact post-surgical outcomes by promoting relaxation, reducing stress, and enhancing the body's healing processes.

Managing Chronic Pain

Chronic pain sufferers have found relief through visualization and imagery techniques. One individual with chronic back pain, unresponsive to conventional treatments, began practicing guided imagery focused on visualizing the pain diminishing and the spine healing. Over time, she reported a significant reduction in pain levels, improved mobility, and a better quality of life. This case illustrates how imagery can reframe the pain experience and mobilize the body's innate healing resources.

Overcoming Performance Anxiety

Performers, including musicians and public speakers, have used visualization to overcome stage fright and enhance performance quality. A concert pianist, for instance, visualized giving flawless performances, focusing on the sensation of her fingers on the keys and the sound of the music, coupled with the feeling of calm and confidence. By mentally rehearsing in this manner, she was able to significantly reduce performance anxiety and improve her concert experiences.

Facilitating Cancer Recovery

In the realm of oncology, visualization techniques have been employed to complement medical treatments for cancer. Patients have visualized their immune cells successfully targeting and destroying cancer cells, alongside their treatments working effectively. Such practices have been associated with improved mood, reduced symptoms of depression and anxiety, and, in some cases, favorable clinical outcomes. While not a substitute for medical treatment, visualization serves as a powerful adjunctive therapy, offering emotional support and potentially enhancing the efficacy of conventional therapies.

Conclusion

These success stories underscore the versatile and powerful role of visualization and imagery in promoting healing, overcoming challenges, and enhancing personal abilities. By harnessing the mind's capacity to influence the body and emotions, individuals can tap into a profound source of strength, resilience, and recovery, highlighting the essential interconnectedness of the mind and body in the healing process.

Guided Imagery Exercises
Step-by-Step Guide

Guided imagery is a relaxation technique that involves visualizing positive images, places, or experiences to bring about relaxation and healing. It leverages the mind-body connection to reduce stress, ease pain, and enhance overall well-being. Here is a step-by-step guide to help you practice guided imagery exercises on your own.

Step 1: Find a Quiet, Comfortable Space

- Preparation: Choose a quiet and comfortable place where you won't be disturbed. Sit or lie down in a comfortable position. You may use cushions or blankets to support your body.

Step 2: Focus on Your Breath

- Initiation: Close your eyes and take a few deep breaths. Inhale slowly through your nose, allowing your belly to rise, and then exhale gently through your mouth. Continue this deep breathing for a few minutes until you feel more relaxed.

Step 3: Enter a Relaxed State

- Deepening Relaxation: To deepen your state of relaxation, perform a quick body scan. Mentally move through different parts of your body, starting from your toes and moving upwards. As you focus on each part, consciously relax and release any tension you find.

Step 4: Visualize Your Peaceful Place

- Imagery Initiation: Imagine a place where you feel completely at ease. This could be a real place you've visited or a fantasy setting. Picture this place in as much detail as possible—the sights, sounds, smells, and textures. For example, if you're imagining a beach, see the turquoise water, hear the waves crashing, smell the salty air, feel the warm sand under your feet.

Step 5: Engage All Your Senses

- Sensory Engagement: Enhance the visualization by engaging all your senses. What do you see around you? What sounds do you hear? Is there a taste or smell associated with this place? What is the texture of the things you might touch? The more senses involved, the more vivid and immersive the experience.

Step 6: Incorporate a Healing Element

- Healing Imagery: If your goal is healing or pain management, introduce an element into your visualization that represents healing or relief. For instance, you might imagine a warm, soothing light enveloping a part of your body that's in pain, gently easing the discomfort.

Step 7: Enjoy the Experience

- Absorption: Allow yourself to fully experience this place and the feelings of relaxation and well-being it brings. Spend several minutes here, soaking in the peace and tranquility.

Step 8: Return to the Present Moment

- Reorientation: When you're ready to finish, slowly bring your awareness back to your physical surroundings. Notice the surface you're sitting or lying on, the temperature of the room, and any sounds around you. Take a few deep breaths.

Step 9: Reflect on the Experience

- Reflection: Before opening your eyes, take a moment to reflect on the experience. How do you feel now compared to before the exercise? Carry this sense of calm and well-being with you as you gently open your eyes and return to your day.

Conclusion

Guided imagery exercises are a powerful tool for promoting relaxation, healing, and emotional well-being. By regularly practicing these steps, you can harness the power of your imagination to positively influence your mind and body, reduce stress, and enhance your quality of life. Remember, like any skill, the benefits of guided imagery grow with practice, so be patient and consistent with your efforts.

Tips for Practice

Enhancing Your Guided Imagery Experience

To maximize the benefits of guided imagery and make your practice more effective and fulfilling, consider these practical tips. Whether you're new to guided imagery or looking to deepen your existing practice, these suggestions can help enhance your experience and foster greater relaxation, healing, and well-being.

1. Regular Practice

- Consistency is Key: Like any skill, the benefits of guided imagery increase with regular practice. Try to incorporate it into your daily routine, even if only for a few minutes at a time.

2. Personalize Your Imagery

- Make It Yours: Tailor your visualizations to reflect your personal preferences, interests, and goals. The more meaningful and resonant your imagery, the more impactful the practice will be.

3. Use Recorded Guides Initially

- Leverage Resources: When starting out, guided imagery recordings can be incredibly helpful. They provide structure and can introduce you to various techniques and scenarios. Over time, you may develop the confidence to guide yourself.

4. Create a Conducive Environment

- Set the Scene: Your physical environment can significantly influence your ability to relax and immerse yourself in the imagery. Find a quiet, comfortable space where you're unlikely to be interrupted. Consider using headphones to block out distractions if you're using a recording.

5. Incorporate Relaxation Techniques

- Relax Your Body: Begin each session with relaxation techniques such as deep breathing or progressive muscle relaxation. A relaxed body can help quiet the mind, making it easier to engage with your imagery.

6. Be Patient and Open-Minded

- Allow the Process to Unfold: Some days, it might be easier to visualize than others. Be patient with yourself and maintain an open-minded attitude toward your practice. Remember, there's no "right" way to experience guided imagery.

7. Keep a Journal

- Reflect on Your Experience: After each session, consider jotting down a few notes about your experience. What imagery did you use? How did it make you feel? Tracking your practice can offer insights into what works best for you and how your experiences evolve over time.

8. Experiment with Different Times of Day

- Find Your Ideal Time: Some people find guided imagery most effective in the morning, setting a positive tone for the day. Others prefer the evening as a way to unwind before sleep. Experiment to find what timing works best for you.

9. Address Distractions

- Manage Intrusive Thoughts: It's normal for the mind to wander during guided imagery. When you notice distractions, gently acknowledge them and redirect your focus back to your visualization without judgment.

10. Combine with Other Practices

- Integrate with Holistic Approaches: Guided imagery can be effectively combined with other practices such as meditation, yoga, or mindfulness. Integrating these techniques can enhance your overall well-being and provide a more comprehensive approach to relaxation and healing.

Conclusion

Guided imagery is a flexible, powerful tool for promoting mental and physical health. By adopting these tips for practice, you can enhance the effectiveness of your guided imagery sessions, making them a more integral and rewarding part of your wellness routine. With patience, consistency, and openness, you can unlock the full potential of guided imagery to foster relaxation, healing, and a deeper connection to your inner self.

Chapter 6: The Power of Emotion

Emotional Regulation and Health

Emotional regulation refers to the processes by which individuals influence which emotions they experience, when they experience them, and how these emotions are expressed. Effective emotional regulation is crucial for mental and physical health, as it affects how people respond to stressors in their environment and manage their internal emotional states.

The Impact of Emotional Regulation on Health:

- Stress Reduction: Proper emotional regulation can lower stress levels. Chronic stress is linked to numerous health issues, including heart disease, diabetes, and weakened immune function. By managing emotional responses to stress, individuals can mitigate these health risks.
- Improved Immune Function: Emotional regulation influences the immune system. Negative emotional states can suppress immune response, while positive emotions and effective emotional management can enhance it, promoting overall health and resilience to illness.
- Mental Health: Emotional dysregulation is a key component of many mental health disorders, such as depression, anxiety, and PTSD. Learning to effectively regulate emotions can help prevent the onset or worsening of these conditions.
- Social Relationships: Emotional regulation skills contribute to healthier and more fulfilling social relationships. The ability to manage emotions effectively can lead to better communication, empathy, and conflict resolution skills, which in turn support social well-being and reduce the emotional stress associated with interpersonal difficulties.

Understanding Emotions

Understanding emotions involves recognizing the complex interplay between feelings, thoughts, and physical reactions within the body. Emotions are not merely psychological phenomena; they have profound physiological effects and can significantly impact health.

Components of Emotions:

- Subjective Experience: The personal, internal experience of emotion is unique to each individual and influenced by personal history, temperament, and the context in which the emotion occurs.
- Physiological Response: Emotions trigger specific physiological responses, such as changes in heart rate, blood pressure, and hormone levels. These responses prepare the body to react to various situations, from fighting off a threat to embracing a loved one.
- Cognitive Appraisal: The way individuals interpret and think about an emotional experience can significantly affect the intensity and duration of their emotions. Cognitive appraisal involves assessing the significance of an event and its implications for personal well-being.
- Expressive Behavior: Emotions are often accompanied by expressive behaviors, such as facial expressions, body language, and vocal tone. These expressions can communicate feelings to others and influence social interactions.

Enhancing Emotional Understanding and Regulation

- Mindfulness Practices: Mindfulness and meditation can enhance emotional awareness and acceptance, allowing individuals to observe their emotions without judgment and respond more thoughtfully.
- Cognitive-Behavioral Techniques: CBT and related therapies can help individuals identify and challenge unhelpful thought patterns that exacerbate emotional distress, promoting healthier emotional regulation.
- Physical Activity: Regular exercise can improve mood, reduce stress, and help regulate emotions through the release of endorphins and the regulation of stress hormones.
- Social Support: Engaging with a supportive social network can provide emotional comfort and validation, facilitating better emotional regulation and resilience.

Conclusion

The power of emotion on health is undeniable, influencing everything from stress levels and immune function to social relationships and mental well-being. By understanding and effectively regulating emotions, individuals can enhance their emotional health, navigate life's challenges more successfully, and foster overall well-being. Through practices such as mindfulness, cognitive-behavioral strategies, and fostering social connections, individuals can develop the skills necessary to manage their emotions and lead healthier, more fulfilling lives.

The Connection Between Heart and Mind

Heart Coherence

The connection between the heart and mind is a fascinating aspect of human physiology and psychology, illustrating how emotional and mental states can directly influence cardiovascular functioning. Heart coherence, a concept brought to light by research in the fields of psychology and neurocardiology, describes a harmonious state of functioning between the heart, mind, and emotions, characterized by increased synchronization and efficiency.

Understanding Heart Coherence

Heart coherence occurs when the heart's rhythmic patterns are smooth and ordered, reflecting a state of balance and coordination within the body's systems. This state is often associated with positive emotions, such as gratitude, love, and joy, and is marked by reduced stress, enhanced mental clarity, and improved emotional regulation.

The heart's rhythmic patterns are measured through heart rate variability (HRV), the variation in time intervals between heartbeats. High HRV is indicative of a healthy, responsive cardiovascular system, while low HRV is associated with stress, fatigue, and increased risk of cardiovascular diseases.

The Science Behind Heart Coherence

Research by the HeartMath Institute and others has shown that heart coherence can be intentionally cultivated through specific practices that evoke positive emotions and promote relaxation. These practices lead to increased synchronization between the heart's rhythms and other bodily systems, including the brain, resulting in:

- Improved Cognitive Functioning: Heart coherence is associated with enhanced concentration, decision-making, and problem-solving abilities.
- Emotional Stability: By promoting a state of inner balance and calm, heart coherence can reduce anxiety, depression, and emotional reactivity.
- Stress Reduction: Heart coherence techniques help downregulate the body's stress response, reducing cortisol levels and mitigating the adverse effects of stress on the body.
- Enhanced Immune Function: The state of coherence has been linked to improved immune system responses, likely due to its stress-reducing effects.

Techniques to Achieve Heart Coherence

1. Focused Breathing: Slow, rhythmic breathing can help shift the body into a state of coherence. Aim for about five to six breaths per minute, focusing on deep, even inhalations and exhalations.
2. Positive Emotion Visualization: Visualize or recall a positive, joyful experience, focusing on the emotions it evokes. Engaging with positive emotions can facilitate the shift into heart coherence.
3. Mindfulness and Meditation: Practices that encourage present-moment awareness and emotional regulation can promote heart coherence by reducing stress and enhancing emotional well-being.
4. Gratitude Practices: Regularly expressing gratitude, either through journaling or mental reflection, can induce heart coherence by fostering positive emotional states.

Conclusion

The connection between the heart and mind, particularly through the concept of heart coherence, offers a compelling insight into how emotional and mental well-being can directly affect physical health. By employing techniques to achieve heart coherence, individuals can enhance their emotional regulation, reduce stress, and promote overall health and well-being, illustrating the profound interconnectedness of the human body and the potential for self-regulation and healing.

Emotional States and Physical Health

The intricate link between emotional states and physical health is a key area of exploration in both psychology and medicine. Understanding how emotions can impact physical well-being sheds light on the importance of emotional regulation and positive psychological practices for maintaining overall health. Emotional states, whether positive or negative, can have profound effects on the body, influencing everything from immune function to cardiovascular health.

Impact of Negative Emotions on Physical Health

Negative emotional states, such as stress, anxiety, and depression, can lead to detrimental health outcomes. The mechanisms through which these emotions affect the body include:

- Stress Response: Chronic stress triggers the release of stress hormones like cortisol and adrenaline, which can lead to elevated blood pressure, increased risk of heart disease, and weakened immune response.
- Inflammation: Negative emotions have been linked to increased inflammation in the body, which is a risk factor for a host of diseases, including arthritis, heart disease, and diabetes.
- Immune Function: Prolonged negative emotional states can suppress immune function, making the body more susceptible to infections and slowing down the healing process.
- Behavioral Factors: Negative emotions can also influence health through behavioral pathways. For example, people experiencing depression or stress may adopt unhealthy coping mechanisms, such as smoking, overeating, or neglecting physical activity.

Benefits of Positive Emotions on Physical Health

Conversely, positive emotional states are associated with a range of health benefits, underscoring the power of positive psychology in promoting physical well-being:

- Enhanced Immune Function: Positive emotions and an optimistic outlook have been shown to boost immune response, offering better protection against illness and promoting faster recovery from health challenges.
- Cardiovascular Health: Happiness and positive affect are linked to lower blood pressure, reduced risk of heart disease, and overall better heart health.
- Longevity: Studies have found a correlation between positive psychological well-being and increased lifespan. Individuals with a positive outlook on life tend to live longer and enjoy better health.
- Stress Resilience: Positive emotions can buffer against the negative effects of stress, helping individuals cope more effectively with life's challenges and reducing the physiological wear and tear associated with chronic stress.

Cultivating Positive Emotional States

Recognizing the impact of emotions on physical health, individuals can take proactive steps to cultivate positive emotional states:

- Practice Gratitude: Regularly reflecting on and appreciating the good aspects of life can enhance positive emotions and well-being.
- Foster Social Connections: Strong, positive relationships contribute to emotional and physical health, providing support and reducing feelings of loneliness and isolation.
- Engage in Activities that Bring Joy: Pursuing hobbies, interests, and activities that bring happiness can improve mood and reduce stress.
- Adopt Mindfulness and Meditation: These practices can help manage negative emotions, reduce stress, and promote a sense of calm and well-being.

- Seek Professional Support: For those struggling with negative emotions or mental health issues, seeking help from a mental health professional can be a crucial step towards improving both emotional and physical health.

Conclusion

The connection between emotional states and physical health is undeniable, highlighting the importance of emotional well-being as a fundamental aspect of overall health. By understanding and actively managing emotions, individuals can not only enhance their mental health but also promote physical health, resilience, and longevity.

Techniques for Emotional Healing

Emotional healing is a crucial aspect of overall well-being, addressing the psychological wounds and traumas that can affect physical health, relationships, and quality of life. Various techniques have been developed to facilitate this healing process, each offering unique approaches to managing and resolving emotional pain. Among these, the Emotional Freedom Technique (EFT) stands out for its simplicity, efficacy, and the growing body of research supporting its use.

Emotional Freedom Technique (EFT)

EFT, often referred to as "tapping," is a psychological acupressure technique that combines elements of cognitive therapy with manual stimulation of acupuncture points (acupoints) on the body. Developed in the 1990s by Gary Craig, EFT is based on the premise that negative emotions are caused by disturbances in the body's energy system and that restoring balance to this system can alleviate psychological distress.

How EFT Works

EFT involves tapping with the fingertips on specific meridian points on the head, face, and upper body while focusing on the emotional issue at hand. The process includes the following steps:

1. Identify the Issue: Begin by clearly identifying the specific emotional issue you wish to address. It's important to be as specific as possible to target the technique effectively.

2. Test the Initial Intensity: Assess the intensity of the emotion or distress on a scale from 0 to 10, with 10 being the highest level of intensity. This provides a baseline for measuring progress.

3. The Setup Statement: While continuously tapping on the "karate chop" point (the side of the hand), repeat a setup statement acknowledging the issue and affirming self-acceptance. For example, "Even though I have this [fear of public speaking], I deeply and completely accept myself."

4. Tapping Sequence: Tap about 7 times on each of the following meridian points in sequence: eyebrow, side of the eye, under the eye, under the nose, chin, beginning of the collarbone, under the arm, and top of the head. While tapping, focus on the issue and your feelings about it.

5. Test the Final Intensity: After completing a few rounds of tapping, reassess the intensity level of your distress. Repeat the tapping sequence as needed until the intensity is significantly reduced or eliminated.

Benefits of EFT

- Stress and Anxiety Reduction: EFT has been shown to significantly reduce stress and anxiety levels, offering a quick and accessible way to manage acute emotional distress.
- Pain Management: By addressing the emotional components of pain, EFT can contribute to pain relief and improved pain management.
- Emotional Trauma Healing: EFT can be effective in processing and healing emotional traumas, reducing symptoms of PTSD and emotional reactivity.
- Improved Well-being: Regular use of EFT can enhance emotional resilience, leading to increased well-being and reduced vulnerability to emotional disturbances.

Conclusion

Techniques for emotional healing, particularly the Emotional Freedom Technique, offer powerful tools for addressing and resolving emotional pain and distress. By integrating these practices into a holistic approach to well-being, individuals can achieve significant improvements in mental health, emotional resilience, and overall quality of life. EFT, with its simplicity and effectiveness, provides a valuable resource for those seeking to overcome emotional challenges and enhance their emotional and physical well-being.

Healing Through Expressive Arts

Healing through expressive arts incorporates a variety of creative modalities, such as painting, drawing, music, dance, drama, and writing, as therapeutic tools to facilitate emotional healing, self-expression, and personal growth. This approach is grounded in the belief that the creative process inherent in artistic self-expression can help individuals explore and resolve emotional issues, reduce stress, and improve psychological well-being.

Principles of Healing Through Expressive Arts

- Self-Expression: Expressive arts provide a non-verbal language for emotions and experiences that may be difficult to articulate with words. This form of expression can reveal unconscious thoughts and feelings, offering new insights and perspectives.
- Mind-Body Connection: Engaging in artistic activities can induce a meditative-like state, promoting relaxation and reducing the physiological effects of stress. This connection between creative expression and physical relaxation underscores the holistic nature of expressive arts therapy.

- Empowerment and Agency: Creating art allows individuals to take control of their healing process, fostering a sense of empowerment and self-efficacy. Completing a piece of art can also provide a sense of accomplishment and boost self-esteem.

How Expressive Arts Promote Healing

1. Enhancing Emotional Regulation: Artistic expression provides an outlet for processing and managing emotions, facilitating emotional release and catharsis. This release can help individuals achieve a more balanced emotional state and improve their capacity for emotional regulation.

2. Reducing Symptoms of Anxiety and Depression: Participation in expressive arts has been shown to decrease symptoms of anxiety and depression, offering a constructive way to cope with negative emotions and mood states.

3. Processing Trauma: For those who have experienced trauma, expressive arts offer a safe medium to explore and express feelings related to traumatic events, aiding in the processing and integration of traumatic memories.

4. Improving Social Connections: Group-based expressive arts activities can enhance social skills and provide a sense of community and belonging. Sharing art and experiences with others can lead to increased empathy, understanding, and support.

5. Fostering Creativity and Problem-Solving: Engaging in the arts stimulates creativity and encourages innovative thinking, which can translate to improved problem-solving skills in other areas of life.

Techniques and Practices

- Art Therapy: Involves using drawing, painting, or sculpting to express and explore emotions, under the guidance of a trained art therapist.
- Music Therapy: Utilizes music listening, songwriting, or playing instruments as a means to address emotional, cognitive, and social needs.
- Dance/Movement Therapy: Uses body movement as a form of expression and communication to promote emotional, mental, and physical integration.
- Writing: Journaling, poetry, or narrative writing can be therapeutic tools for reflecting on personal experiences and expressing emotions.
- Drama Therapy: Involves role-play, storytelling, and theatrical performances as methods for exploring personal stories and emotional conflicts.

Conclusion

Healing through expressive arts offers a unique and powerful avenue for addressing emotional and psychological challenges. By facilitating self-expression, enhancing emotional regulation, and fostering a sense of empowerment, expressive arts therapies contribute to overall well-being and resilience. Whether practiced independently or with the support of a therapist, the creative process inherent in these modalities provides a valuable resource for personal growth and healing.

Chapter 7: Lifestyle Factors in Self-Healing

Nutrition and Healing

Nutrition plays a pivotal role in the body's self-healing processes, offering the necessary building blocks for repair, supporting immune function, and reducing inflammation. A balanced, nutrient-rich diet can significantly influence recovery times, resilience against illness, and overall well-being. Understanding the connection between nutrition and healing provides a foundation for making dietary choices that support health and recovery.

Foods That Promote Healing

1. Whole Fruits and Vegetables

- Benefits: Rich in vitamins, minerals, antioxidants, and fiber, fruits and vegetables combat oxidative stress and inflammation, key factors in many chronic diseases and the healing process.
- Examples: Berries, leafy greens, cruciferous vegetables (broccoli, Brussels sprouts), and bright-colored fruits (oranges, mangoes).

2. Lean Proteins

- Benefits: Proteins are essential for tissue repair and immune function. Lean sources provide the necessary amino acids for healing without excessive saturated fat.
- Examples: Poultry, fish, beans, lentils, and tofu.

3. Healthy Fats

- Benefits: Fats are crucial for cell membrane integrity and hormone production. Omega-3 fatty acids, in particular, have anti-inflammatory properties that can aid in healing.
- Examples: Fatty fish (salmon, mackerel), avocados, nuts, seeds, and olive oil.

4. Whole Grains

- Benefits: Rich in fiber, whole grains help maintain a healthy gut microbiome, which is vital for immune function and inflammation regulation.
- Examples: Quinoa, brown rice, oats, and barley.

5. Probiotic and Prebiotic Foods

- Benefits: Probiotics support gut health and immunity, while prebiotics feed beneficial gut bacteria, promoting a healthy digestive system.
- Examples: Yogurt, kefir (probiotics); garlic, onions, bananas (prebiotics).

6. Herbs and Spices

- Benefits: Many herbs and spices have potent anti-inflammatory and antioxidant properties, offering additional support for the body's healing processes.
- Examples: Turmeric (curcumin), ginger, cinnamon, and garlic.

7. Hydration

- Benefits: Adequate hydration is essential for all bodily functions, including the efficient removal of toxins and the optimal function of the immune system.
- Recommendation: Drink plenty of water throughout the day, and consider hydrating foods like cucumbers and watermelon.

Integrating Healing Foods into Your Diet

- Variety and Balance: Incorporate a wide range of healing foods into your diet to ensure you're getting a broad spectrum of nutrients. Aim for a colorful plate at each meal to maximize nutrient intake.
- Mindful Eating: Pay attention to your body's hunger and fullness cues, and eat with mindfulness to support digestion and nutrient absorption.
- Preparation Methods: Opt for cooking methods that preserve the nutrient content and natural flavors of foods, such as steaming, baking, or sautéing, rather than frying.

Conclusion

Nutrition is a cornerstone of self-healing, with the power to influence the body's repair mechanisms, immune response, and overall resilience. By prioritizing healing foods and adopting a mindful approach to eating, individuals can support their body's natural healing processes, enhance their health, and prevent disease. This holistic approach to nutrition underscores the integral role of dietary choices in maintaining health and facilitating recovery.

Anti-inflammatory Diet

An anti-inflammatory diet focuses on consuming foods that reduce inflammation in the body, a critical factor in preventing and managing a wide range of chronic diseases, including heart disease, diabetes, arthritis, and certain cancers. Chronic inflammation is also linked to aging and conditions such as obesity. By emphasizing nutrient-dense, whole foods and minimizing the intake of processed foods and inflammatory agents, an anti-inflammatory diet can support the body's healing processes, enhance overall health, and improve quality of life.

Key Components of an Anti-inflammatory Diet

1. Fruits and Vegetables: Rich in antioxidants and phytochemicals, fruits and vegetables can reduce oxidative stress and inflammation. Focus on a variety of colors to maximize the range of protective compounds consumed.
   - *Examples:* Berries, cherries, apples, oranges, leafy greens, and cruciferous vegetables like broccoli and Brussels sprouts.

2. Whole Grains: Whole grains contain fiber, which can help reduce C-reactive protein (a marker of inflammation) in the blood.
   - *Examples:* Oats, brown rice, quinoa, and whole wheat.

3. Healthy Fats: Omega-3 fatty acids, found in certain types of fish and other sources, are known for their anti-inflammatory properties. Monounsaturated fats are also beneficial.
   - *Examples:* Salmon, mackerel, flaxseeds, chia seeds, walnuts, avocados, and extra-virgin olive oil.

4. Nuts and Seeds: These are good sources of anti-inflammatory fats, fiber, and antioxidants.
   - *Examples:* Almonds, walnuts, flaxseeds, and chia seeds.

5. Legumes: High in fiber, protein, and antioxidants, legumes can help combat inflammation.
   - *Examples:* Beans, lentils, and chickpeas.

6. Herbs and Spices: Many herbs and spices contain compounds that offer powerful anti-inflammatory effects.
   - *Examples:* Turmeric (curcumin), ginger, garlic, and cinnamon.

7. Tea: Green tea, in particular, is rich in epigallocatechin gallate (EGCG), a compound with strong anti-inflammatory properties.

Foods to Avoid

Reducing or eliminating foods known to contribute to inflammation can enhance the benefits of an anti-inflammatory diet. These include:

- Processed and Refined Foods: High in additives and low in nutrients, processed foods can trigger inflammatory responses.
- Sugar and High-fructose Corn Syrup: Excessive consumption of sugar and sweeteners can lead to increased inflammation.
- Trans Fats: Found in some processed and fried foods, trans fats are strongly linked to inflammation and heart disease.
- Excessive Alcohol: While moderate consumption may have some health benefits, excessive alcohol intake is associated with inflammation.

Implementing an Anti-inflammatory Diet

- Gradual Changes: Incorporate more anti-inflammatory foods into your diet gradually, replacing processed foods with whole, nutrient-dense options.
- Hydration: Drinking plenty of water helps flush toxins from the body, supporting the anti-inflammatory diet's effects.
- Balance: Ensure your diet is balanced and diverse to cover all essential nutrients, vitamins, and minerals.

Conclusion

An anti-inflammatory diet is not just about reducing inflammation; it's a holistic approach to eating that emphasizes nutritious foods for overall health. By focusing on whole foods and minimizing intake of processed items and inflammatory agents, individuals can significantly impact their health, reduce disease risk, and promote longevity. As with any dietary change, it's beneficial to consult with a healthcare professional or a registered dietitian to tailor the approach to your specific health needs and conditions.

Exercise and the Mind-Body Connection: Physical Activity as Medicine

Exercise is widely recognized not only for its physical health benefits but also for its profound impact on mental and emotional well-being. This dual influence underscores the deep connection between the mind and body, highlighting the role of physical activity as a form of medicine that can heal, energize, and balance the human system.

Exercise and the Mind-Body Connection

The mind-body connection in exercise is evident in how physical activity can influence mental states, emotional regulation, and overall psychological health. Regular exercise has been shown to:

- Reduce Stress: Physical activity increases the production of endorphins, the body's natural mood elevators, which can reduce stress levels and elevate mood.
- Enhance Cognitive Function: Exercise can improve cognitive function across the lifespan, contributing to better memory, attention, and executive function. It stimulates the production of growth factors that enhance neural health and plasticity.
- Improve Sleep Quality: By promoting physical tiredness and reducing stress and anxiety, exercise can lead to better sleep quality and duration, further supporting mental health.
- Boost Self-esteem and Confidence: Achieving exercise goals or milestones, no matter how small, can improve self-esteem and body image, fostering a more positive self-concept.

Physical Activity as Medicine

Viewing physical activity as medicine involves recognizing its role in preventing and managing chronic diseases, improving physical health markers, and enhancing quality of life. Key aspects include:

- Disease Prevention and Management: Regular exercise can help prevent the onset of chronic diseases such as heart disease, diabetes, obesity, and certain types of cancer. For those already managing chronic conditions, physical activity can improve symptoms and reduce the severity of the disease.
- Physical Rehabilitation and Recovery: Exercise is a critical component of rehabilitation programs for injuries and surgeries. Tailored physical activity can speed recovery, restore function, and prevent complications.
- Pain Management: For chronic pain conditions, exercise can be an effective management strategy. It helps strengthen muscles, increase flexibility, and reduce the intensity and frequency of pain episodes.

- Longevity and Healthy Aging: Regular physical activity is associated with increased lifespan and improved quality of life in older adults. It supports healthy aging by maintaining physical function, preventing falls, and enhancing cognitive health.

Implementing Exercise as a Therapeutic Tool

- Consult Healthcare Providers: Before starting any new exercise regimen, especially for individuals with existing health conditions, it's important to consult with healthcare professionals to design a safe and effective program.
- Find Enjoyable Activities: Exercise should be enjoyable to ensure long-term engagement. Exploring different types of activities, such as walking, cycling, swimming, yoga, or team sports, can help identify what feels best.
- Set Realistic Goals: Setting achievable, realistic goals can help maintain motivation and provide a sense of accomplishment.
- Incorporate Mindfulness: Engaging in exercise mindfully, paying attention to the body's movements and sensations during physical activity, can enhance the mind-body connection and increase the therapeutic benefits of exercise.

Conclusion

The relationship between exercise and the mind-body connection is a powerful testament to the role of physical activity in achieving and maintaining holistic health. By approaching exercise as a form of medicine, individuals can leverage its comprehensive benefits to improve physical, mental, and emotional well-being, embodying the true essence of a mind-body approach to health and healing.

Types of Exercise for Mental Health

Physical activity is a powerful tool for enhancing mental health, with various types of exercise offering unique benefits for reducing stress, anxiety, depression, and improving overall emotional well-being. Tailoring exercise to individual preferences and mental health goals can maximize these benefits, making physical activity an integral part of a holistic mental health strategy.

1. Aerobic Exercise

- Description: Aerobic exercise, also known as cardio, involves continuous, rhythmic physical activity that increases heart rate and breath. It includes walking, running, cycling, swimming, and dancing.
- Mental Health Benefits: Aerobic exercise has been extensively studied for its positive effects on mental health, including reducing symptoms of depression and anxiety, improving mood, and increasing levels of endorphins and neurotransmitters like serotonin and dopamine that contribute to feelings of well-being.

2. Strength Training

- Description: Strength training, or resistance training, involves exercises that improve muscular strength and endurance, using weights, resistance bands, or body weight.

- Mental Health Benefits: Engaging in regular strength training can alleviate symptoms of depression, enhance self-esteem, and improve cognitive function. It also provides a sense of accomplishment and can be a productive outlet for stress and frustration.

3. Yoga

- Description: Yoga combines physical postures, breath control, and meditation to enhance physical flexibility, strength, and mental relaxation.
- Mental Health Benefits: Yoga is particularly beneficial for reducing stress, anxiety, and symptoms of depression. Its meditative aspect can enhance mindfulness, emotional balance, and overall sense of peace.

4. Tai Chi and Qigong

- Description: Tai Chi and Qigong are forms of gentle martial arts combining slow, deliberate movements, meditation, and breath control to promote physical and mental well-being.
- Mental Health Benefits: These practices are known for reducing stress, improving mood, and enhancing mental clarity. They are particularly suitable for individuals seeking low-impact exercise that fosters a sense of calm and balance.

5. High-Intensity Interval Training (HIIT)

- Description: HIIT consists of short bursts of intense exercise followed by periods of rest or low-intensity exercise. It's a time-efficient way to exercise and can include activities like sprinting, jumping, or circuit training.
- Mental Health Benefits: HIIT has been shown to quickly improve mood, reduce stress, and can be particularly effective for those with busy schedules, offering a quick mental "reset."

6. Outdoor Activities

- Description: Outdoor activities like hiking, biking, or even gardening offer the dual benefits of exercise and nature exposure, which have been shown to have synergistic effects on mental health.
- Mental Health Benefits: Being in nature while exercising can enhance mood, decrease stress, and improve feelings of vitality and energy. The natural setting can also improve attention and reduce symptoms of mental fatigue.

7. Team Sports

- Description: Participating in team sports such as soccer, basketball, or volleyball involves both physical activity and social interaction.
- Mental Health Benefits: Team sports can reduce feelings of isolation, build social support networks, and improve mood and self-esteem through both the physical activity and the sense of community and belonging they foster.

Conclusion

The diverse range of exercises suitable for enhancing mental health highlights the importance of incorporating physical activity into mental health care. Whether seeking the meditative calm of yoga, the endorphin boost of aerobic exercise, or the social support of team sports, individuals can find activities that resonate with their personal preferences and mental health needs. Regular engagement in these activities can significantly contribute to improved mental well-being, demonstrating the powerful role of exercise in supporting mental health.

Sleep and Recovery: The Science of Sleep

Sleep plays a crucial role in physical and mental recovery, serving as a foundational pillar of health alongside nutrition and exercise. Understanding the science of sleep reveals its complex functions in healing, restoration, and cognitive processing, highlighting the importance of quality sleep for overall well-being and effective recovery from daily stressors and physical exertion.

The Functions of Sleep

Sleep is not merely a passive state of rest but an active period of physiological and psychological restoration. Its critical functions include:

- Physical Repair and Growth: During sleep, the body undergoes repair and growth processes, facilitated by the release of growth hormone. This includes muscle repair, tissue growth, and protein synthesis, essential for recovery from physical activity and injury.
- Immune System Strengthening: Sleep enhances immune function. Adequate sleep can improve the body's ability to fend off infections and diseases by optimizing immune response.
- Cognitive Processing and Memory Consolidation: Sleep plays a vital role in cognitive function, including learning, memory consolidation, and emotional regulation. During sleep, the brain processes and consolidates information from the day, making it crucial for learning and memory retention.
- Detoxification and Brain Health: The glymphatic system, active during sleep, removes toxins from the brain that accumulate during waking hours. This process is essential for maintaining brain health and preventing neurodegenerative diseases.

The Stages of Sleep

Sleep is divided into several stages, each with distinct physiological characteristics and functions:

1. NREM (Non-Rapid Eye Movement) Sleep:
   - *Stage 1:* The transition from wakefulness to sleep, characterized by light sleep and easy awakenings.
   - *Stage 2:* Light sleep preceding deeper sleep; body temperature drops, and heart rate slows.
   - *Stage 3:* Deep sleep stage, crucial for physical recovery and immune function.

2. REM (Rapid Eye Movement) Sleep:
   - Occurs approximately 90 minutes after falling asleep, characterized by rapid eye movements, increased brain activity, vivid dreams, and temporary muscle paralysis. REM sleep is essential for cognitive functions, including memory consolidation and emotional regulation.

The Impact of Sleep Deprivation

Lack of quality sleep can have significant negative effects on health, including:

- Impaired Cognitive Function: Sleep deprivation can lead to decreased attention, impaired memory, and reduced decision-making abilities.
- Emotional and Mental Health Issues: Insufficient sleep is linked to increased risk of depression, anxiety, and mood disorders.
- Physical Health Risks: Chronic sleep deprivation is associated with higher risks of obesity, heart disease, diabetes, and reduced immune function.

Strategies for Improving Sleep Quality

To harness the restorative power of sleep, consider implementing the following strategies:

- Consistent Sleep Schedule: Going to bed and waking up at the same time every day helps regulate the body's internal clock, improving sleep quality.
- Optimizing Sleep Environment: Ensure your sleeping environment is conducive to rest, with comfortable bedding, minimal noise, and cool temperatures.
- Limiting Stimulants: Avoid caffeine and electronic devices close to bedtime, as they can interfere with the ability to fall asleep.
- Relaxation Techniques: Practices such as reading, taking a warm bath, or meditation before bed can help signal to your body that it's time to wind down.

Conclusion

The science of sleep underscores its critical role in health, recovery, and well-being. By prioritizing sleep and adopting habits that enhance sleep quality, individuals can support their body's natural healing processes, improve cognitive function, and maintain overall health. Recognizing sleep as a vital component of recovery strategies emphasizes the need for a holistic approach to health that integrates sleep, nutrition, and physical activity.

Strategies for Better Sleep

Achieving quality sleep is essential for physical health, emotional well-being, and cognitive performance. Implementing effective strategies for better sleep can help overcome common sleep disturbances and ensure restorative rest. Here are practical steps to enhance sleep quality and promote healthy sleep patterns.

1. Establish a Consistent Sleep Schedule

- Routine Matters: Try to go to bed and wake up at the same time every day, even on weekends. Consistency reinforces your body's sleep-wake cycle, making it easier to fall asleep and wake up naturally.

2. Create a Pre-Sleep Ritual

- Wind Down: Develop a relaxing bedtime routine to signal to your body that it's time to wind down. This can include activities like reading, taking a warm bath, or practicing relaxation exercises.

3. Optimize Your Sleep Environment

- Comfort is Key: Ensure your bedroom is conducive to sleep. This means a comfortable mattress and pillows, and a room that's cool, dark, and quiet. Consider using blackout curtains, eye masks, earplugs, or white noise machines if needed.

4. Limit Exposure to Screens

- Reduce Blue Light: The blue light emitted by screens can interfere with your body's ability to produce melatonin, a hormone that regulates sleep. Try to avoid screens at least one hour before bedtime.

5. Watch Your Diet

- Mindful Eating: Avoid heavy or large meals within a couple of hours of bedtime. Be cautious with nicotine, caffeine, and alcohol, as they can disrupt sleep.

6. Exercise Regularly

- Stay Active: Regular physical activity can help you fall asleep faster and enjoy deeper sleep. However, avoid exercising too close to bedtime, as it may increase energy levels and make it harder to fall asleep.

7. Manage Stress

- Relaxation Techniques: Practice stress-reducing techniques such as deep breathing, meditation, or yoga. Managing stress effectively can prevent it from interfering with sleep.

8. Limit Naps

- Nap Wisely: While naps can be a great way to catch up on missed sleep, long or irregular napping during the day can affect nighttime sleep. If you choose to nap, limit it to 20-30 minutes and avoid napping late in the day.

9. Get Natural Light Exposure

- Sunlight Benefits: Exposure to natural light during the day helps regulate sleep patterns. Try to spend time outside or in brightly lit environments during daylight hours.

10. Seek Professional Help if Needed

- Address Sleep Disorders: If you consistently struggle to sleep well and feel it's affecting your daily life, consider seeking help from a healthcare provider. Sleep disorders like insomnia, sleep apnea, and restless legs syndrome require professional evaluation and treatment.

Conclusion

Improving sleep quality involves a combination of lifestyle adjustments, environmental modifications, and possibly medical intervention for underlying sleep disorders. By adopting these strategies for better sleep, individuals can enhance their sleep quality, contributing to improved health, mood, and overall quality of life. Emphasizing the importance of sleep in the broader context of health and well-being is essential for maintaining a balanced and healthy lifestyle.

Chapter 8: Integrative Approaches to Self-Healing

Combining Western and Alternative Medicine

Integrative approaches to self-healing represent a holistic strategy that combines the strengths of Western medicine with alternative and complementary therapies. This approach acknowledges the complex interplay between the physical, emotional, mental, and environmental factors influencing health, aiming to treat the whole person rather than just the symptoms or disease. By blending evidence-based conventional medical treatments with time-tested traditional practices, individuals can access a comprehensive, personalized care plan that promotes healing, well-being, and disease prevention.

Key Principles of Integrative Medicine:

- Patient-Centered Care: Focuses on the patient as a whole person, considering their unique circumstances, needs, and perspectives.
- Evidence-Informed Practices: Utilizes the best available research evidence to guide treatment choices, combining them with clinical expertise and patient preferences.
- Preventive and Holistic Approach: Emphasizes the importance of preventing disease and maintaining health, considering lifestyle, nutrition, stress management, and environmental factors.
- Collaborative Treatment Planning: Involves collaboration between healthcare providers and patients to develop tailored treatment plans that align with the patient's goals and values.

Case Studies of Integrative Healing

Case Study 1: Chronic Pain Management

Background: A patient with chronic lower back pain, unresponsive to conventional pain medications and physical therapy, explores integrative approaches for relief.

Integrative Strategy:
- Western Medicine: Continuation of physical therapy focusing on strengthening and flexibility exercises.
- Alternative Therapies: Introduction of acupuncture and yoga to address pain and improve body mechanics.
- Outcome: The patient experienced significant pain reduction, increased mobility, and improved quality of life, illustrating the benefits of a multi-modal approach to chronic pain management.

Case Study 2: Managing Anxiety and Depression

Background: An individual struggling with anxiety and depression seeks alternatives to pharmacological treatment due to side effects and incomplete relief.

Integrative Strategy:

- Western Medicine: Utilization of psychotherapy to address underlying emotional issues and cognitive patterns contributing to mental health conditions.
- Alternative Therapies: Incorporation of meditation, herbal supplements (under medical supervision), and nutritional counseling to support mental health.
- Outcome: The individual reported improved mood, reduced anxiety levels, and a greater sense of well-being, highlighting the effectiveness of combining psychotherapy with holistic self-care practices.

Case Study 3: Recovery from Surgery

Background: A patient undergoing surgery seeks integrative approaches to enhance recovery and minimize post-operative complications.

Integrative Strategy:
- Western Medicine: Adherence to post-operative care recommendations and medication regimen for pain management and infection prevention.
- Alternative Therapies: Implementation of guided imagery and relaxation techniques to reduce stress and promote healing; nutritional support to optimize recovery.
- Outcome: The patient experienced a faster recovery, reduced pain medication needs, and fewer complications, demonstrating the role of stress management and nutrition in surgical recovery.

Conclusion

Integrative approaches to self-healing offer a comprehensive model of care that combines the best of Western medicine and alternative therapies. By addressing the full spectrum of factors influencing health and well-being, integrative medicine empowers individuals to take an active role in their healing journey, promoting resilience, recovery, and a higher quality of life. These case studies exemplify the potential of integrative healing strategies to provide effective, personalized care that meets the unique needs and preferences of each individual.

How to Choose the Right Approach for Integrative Self-Healing

Navigating the landscape of integrative self-healing can be complex, given the wide array of available Western and alternative therapies. Choosing the right approach involves a thoughtful consideration of your unique health needs, preferences, and goals. Here are steps and considerations to help guide you in selecting the most appropriate and effective integrative healing strategies for you.

1. Assess Your Health Needs

- Identify Specific Health Concerns: Begin by clearly identifying your health issues, symptoms, and conditions that you wish to address. This could range from chronic pain, mental health challenges, lifestyle diseases, to general wellness goals.
- Understand Your Body: Consider any personal health factors that might influence your choice of therapies, such as allergies, sensitivities, or pre-existing conditions.

2. Research and Educate Yourself

- Learn About Options: Research both conventional and alternative therapies that are commonly used for your specific health concerns. Look for evidence-based information to understand the benefits, risks, and effectiveness of each option.
- Seek Reliable Sources: Utilize reputable sources such as academic journals, healthcare organizations, and trusted wellness platforms for your research.

3. Consult Healthcare Professionals

- Seek Expert Advice: Consult with healthcare providers, including your primary care physician and specialists in both conventional and alternative medicine. They can offer professional insights into your health condition and recommend appropriate treatment options.
- Consider Integrative Medicine Practitioners: Specialists in integrative medicine can provide guidance on combining therapies effectively and safely.

4. Evaluate Safety and Evidence

- Safety First: Assess the safety of potential therapies, especially in relation to your health status and any other treatments you may be receiving. Be cautious of treatments with significant risks or those that advise against conventional medical advice.
- Evidence of Effectiveness: Prioritize therapies with strong evidence for effectiveness in treating your specific conditions or meeting your wellness goals.

5. Reflect on Personal Preferences and Lifestyle

- Personal Compatibility: Consider your preferences, lifestyle, and values. Some therapies may align better with your personal beliefs and daily routine, enhancing your commitment and the therapy's effectiveness.
- Practical Considerations: Take into account factors such as cost, accessibility, and time commitment required for each therapy option.

6. Trial and Monitoring

- Start Small: Begin with one or a few therapies that seem most promising and compatible with your needs. Avoid overwhelming yourself with too many changes at once.
- Monitor Progress: Keep track of your health and well-being as you try new therapies. Note any improvements, side effects, or changes in symptoms.

7. Adjust Based on Experience

- Be Flexible: Be prepared to adjust your approach based on your experiences and outcomes. Healing is a dynamic process, and what works best may evolve over time.
- Ongoing Communication with Healthcare Providers: Maintain open lines of communication with your healthcare providers, informing them of all the therapies you are using and any changes in your health.

Conclusion

Choosing the right approach for integrative self-healing requires a combination of self-awareness, thorough research, professional guidance, and mindful experimentation. By carefully considering your unique health needs, the available evidence, and your personal preferences, you can develop a tailored integrative healing plan that supports your journey toward health and well-being. Remember, the most effective approach is one that respects the interconnectedness of your physical, mental, and emotional health, aligning with your lifestyle and goals.

Acupuncture, Massage, and Other Therapies
Overview of Alternative Therapies

Alternative therapies encompass a wide range of practices that fall outside the realm of conventional Western medicine. These therapies, often rooted in ancient traditions, offer diverse approaches to healing, focusing on the body, mind, and spirit's interconnectedness. Among these, acupuncture and massage therapy stand out for their widespread use and growing acceptance within integrative health care. This overview explores these and other alternative therapies, shedding light on their principles, applications, and potential benefits for health and well-being.

Acupuncture

- Principles: Acupuncture is a key component of Traditional Chinese Medicine (TCM) that involves the insertion of thin needles into specific points on the body, known as acupuncture points. It is based on the concept of Qi (vital energy) flowing through meridians (energy pathways) in the body. Acupuncture aims to restore balance and encourage the body's natural healing response by stimulating these points.
- Applications: It is used to treat a variety of conditions, including pain relief, stress management, anxiety, depression, and digestive disorders. Acupuncture is also utilized for enhancing general wellness and preventing illness.
- Evidence and Acceptance: Numerous studies support acupuncture's efficacy, particularly in pain management and for nausea related to chemotherapy or surgery. Its acceptance in Western countries has grown, with many health practitioners referring patients for acupuncture alongside conventional treatments.

Massage Therapy

- Principles: Massage therapy involves manipulating the body's soft tissues (muscles, connective tissues, tendons, ligaments) through various techniques to promote relaxation, healing, and well-being. It works by relieving muscle tension, improving circulation, and reducing stress levels.
- Applications: Massage is beneficial for relieving stress, anxiety, muscle pain, stiffness, and improving sleep quality. It is often used in sports medicine to aid recovery from injuries and enhance athletic performance.
- Evidence and Acceptance: Research supports massage therapy's benefits for various conditions, including chronic low-back pain, neck pain, and tension headaches. Massage is widely accepted and often integrated into holistic health programs and rehabilitation.

Other Alternative Therapies

- Yoga: Combines physical postures, breath control, and meditation to enhance flexibility, strength, and mental calmness. Yoga has been shown to reduce stress, improve mental health, and support physical wellness.

- Meditation: Involves practices focused on developing mindfulness, concentration, and emotional balance. Meditation can reduce symptoms of anxiety and depression, improve attention, and contribute to a sense of peace.

- Chiropractic Care: Focuses on diagnosing and treating musculoskeletal disorders, particularly those involving the spine. Chiropractic adjustments aim to restore joint function, alleviate pain, and support the body's natural healing abilities.

- Herbal Medicine: Uses plants and plant extracts to treat various health conditions. Herbal remedies can support health holistically, but they require careful consideration for safety and interactions with conventional medications.

- Reiki: A form of energy healing where practitioners seek to facilitate the patient's process of healing through what is described as universal energy. It aims to promote relaxation, reduce stress, and foster a healing environment.

Conclusion

Alternative therapies offer a broad spectrum of approaches to health and healing, emphasizing the body's inherent ability to heal and maintain balance. Acupuncture, massage therapy, and other practices provide valuable tools for individuals seeking holistic approaches to health care, often complementing conventional medical treatments. As interest in integrative health continues to grow, these therapies gain recognition for their potential to enhance well-being, manage symptoms, and improve quality of life. It's essential, however, to approach these therapies with informed knowledge and in consultation with healthcare professionals to ensure their safe and effective use.

What the Research Says: Efficacy of Alternative Therapies

The efficacy of alternative therapies has been a subject of growing interest and research within the medical and scientific communities. As the demand for holistic and integrative health approaches increases, understanding what research says about the effectiveness of these therapies is crucial for informed health care decisions. This overview examines the current state of research on several key alternative therapies, highlighting their potential benefits and limitations based on scientific evidence.

Acupuncture

Research on acupuncture has shown it to be effective for certain conditions, especially for pain management and nausea. Systematic reviews and meta-analyses have found acupuncture to be beneficial in treating chronic pain conditions such as lower back pain, neck pain, and osteoarthritis knee pain. Additionally, acupuncture has been shown to reduce the frequency and intensity of tension headaches and migraines. The World Health Organization (WHO) also recognizes acupuncture as effective for over two dozen conditions, including hypertension and allergic rhinitis.

Massage Therapy

Massage therapy has been extensively studied for its effects on pain, stress, and muscle tension. Research indicates that massage therapy can significantly reduce pain in conditions like postoperative pain, fibromyalgia, and low back pain. Massage is also effective in reducing stress and improving mood, making it a beneficial treatment for anxiety and depression. Furthermore, massage may enhance immune function by increasing the activity of natural killer cells and lymphocytes.

Yoga

Yoga's benefits for physical and mental health are supported by a growing body of research. Studies have shown that regular yoga practice can improve cardiovascular health by lowering blood pressure and heart rate, enhance respiratory function, and reduce chronic pain. Yoga has also been found to alleviate symptoms of anxiety, depression, and stress, likely due to its emphasis on mindfulness and relaxation. Moreover, yoga can improve quality of life and well-being in various populations, including cancer survivors and individuals with chronic diseases.

Meditation

Meditation, particularly mindfulness meditation, has been the focus of considerable research. Findings suggest that meditation can reduce symptoms of anxiety and depression, improve attention and concentration, and decrease stress levels. Neuroimaging studies have revealed that meditation can lead to structural changes in areas of the brain associated with attention, emotional regulation, and self-awareness. Meditation practices are increasingly incorporated into psychological therapies, such as Mindfulness-Based Stress Reduction (MBSR) and Mindfulness-Based Cognitive Therapy (MBCT), for their mental health benefits.

Herbal Medicine

The effectiveness of herbal medicine varies widely depending on the herb, condition being treated, and quality of the product. Some herbs have been well-studied and found to be effective for specific conditions. For example, St. John's Wort has shown efficacy in treating mild to moderate depression, and Ginkgo Biloba may improve cognitive function in individuals with dementia. However, the variability in herbal product quality and potential interactions with conventional medications highlight the need for cautious use and professional guidance.

Conclusion

The research on alternative therapies demonstrates their potential as complementary treatments for a range of physical and mental health conditions. While evidence supports the efficacy of therapies like acupuncture, massage, yoga, and meditation for specific health outcomes, the effectiveness of herbal medicine and other alternative practices may vary. It is essential for individuals to consult healthcare professionals when considering alternative therapies, ensuring treatments are evidence-based, safe, and appropriate for their health needs. As research continues to evolve, it will further illuminate the role of alternative therapies in holistic health care and integrative medicine practices.

Creating Your Personal Healing Plan: Assessing Your Needs

Developing a personal healing plan is a proactive approach to enhancing your health and well-being, addressing both physical and emotional aspects of healing. The first critical step in this process is assessing your needs, which lays the foundation for a tailored plan that resonates with your unique health situation, preferences, and goals. This assessment involves introspection, honesty, and sometimes, professional guidance to identify areas requiring attention and to determine the most effective strategies for improvement.

Steps for Assessing Your Needs

1. Reflect on Your Physical Health:
   - Evaluate any existing health conditions, chronic pain, or physical discomfort you may be experiencing.
   - Consider your energy levels, sleep quality, and any symptoms that impact your daily life.

2. Consider Your Emotional and Mental Well-being:
   - Assess your stress levels, emotional balance, and any feelings of anxiety or depression.
   - Reflect on your coping mechanisms for stress and whether they are healthy and effective.

3. Examine Your Lifestyle:
   - Look at your diet, physical activity levels, and relaxation practices. Are they supporting your health and well-being?
   - Consider your work-life balance and how your daily routines contribute to or detract from your health.

4. Identify Your Health Goals:
   - Set clear, achievable health goals based on your assessment. These might include improving sleep quality, reducing stress, managing a health condition more effectively, or enhancing overall physical fitness.

5. Review Your Support System:
   - Consider the role of social support in your healing journey. Do you have access to supportive friends, family, or community resources?
   - Think about whether you might benefit from professional support, such as counseling, a dietitian, or a fitness coach.

Creating a Balanced Healing Plan

Once you've assessed your needs, you can begin to create a balanced, comprehensive healing plan that addresses physical health, emotional well-being, lifestyle factors, and support systems. Your plan might include:

- Physical Health Strategies: Such as specific medical treatments for existing conditions, complementary therapies (e.g., acupuncture, massage), or a targeted exercise regimen.

- Emotional and Mental Health Approaches: Incorporating practices like mindfulness, meditation, or therapy to manage stress, anxiety, or depression.

- Lifestyle Modifications: Adjusting your diet to include more nutrient-rich foods, setting a consistent sleep schedule, and finding hobbies or activities that bring you joy and relaxation.

- Building a Support Network: Engaging more with friends and family or seeking out community groups with similar health goals or experiences. Consider professional guidance for personalized support.

Conclusion

Assessing your needs is a crucial first step in creating a personal healing plan that addresses your unique health challenges and goals. By taking a holistic view of your health and well-being, you can develop a plan that not only focuses on treating symptoms but also promotes overall health, happiness, and quality of life. Remember, your healing plan can evolve over time as your needs change, so revisit and adjust it as necessary to continue supporting your journey toward health and well-being.

Setting Goals and Tracking Progress in Your Personal Healing Plan

After assessing your needs, the next step in creating an effective personal healing plan involves setting clear, achievable goals and establishing a system to track your progress. This approach ensures that your plan is focused, measurable, and adaptable, allowing you to stay motivated and make informed adjustments as needed.

Setting SMART Goals

SMART goals—Specific, Measurable, Achievable, Relevant, and Time-bound—provide a framework for creating objectives that are clear and attainable. Applying this framework to your health goals can enhance your chances of success.

- Specific: Define what you want to achieve with as much detail as possible. Instead of "get healthy," aim for "reduce my blood sugar levels to within the normal range."
- Measurable: Ensure your goal can be tracked and measured. For example, "walk 30 minutes a day, five days a week."
- Achievable: Set goals that are realistic and attainable, considering your current health, resources, and constraints.

- Relevant: Choose goals that are meaningful and important to you, aligning with your broader health and well-being aspirations.
- Time-bound: Set a timeframe for achieving your goal to maintain focus and motivation, such as "within the next three months."

Tracking Progress

Consistent tracking of your progress helps maintain motivation, provides insights into what's working or not, and allows for timely adjustments to your plan.

- Journaling: Keep a health journal to document your activities, symptoms, emotional states, and any changes you notice. This record can reveal patterns and progress over time.
- Digital Tools: Use apps or digital health trackers to monitor specific health metrics related to your goals, such as sleep quality, physical activity, or dietary intake.
- Check-ins: Schedule regular check-ins with yourself (and possibly with a healthcare provider or coach) to review your progress, celebrate achievements, and address challenges.
- Adaptability: Be prepared to adjust your goals and strategies based on your progress and any new information. Flexibility is key to a successful healing journey.

Celebrating Milestones

Recognizing and celebrating milestones, no matter how small, can boost your confidence and motivation. Set mini-goals within your broader objectives and reward yourself for achieving them.

Conclusion

Setting SMART goals and tracking your progress are essential components of a personal healing plan. They provide direction, motivation, and a framework for evaluating the effectiveness of your strategies. By remaining committed to your goals, regularly assessing your progress, and being willing to make necessary adjustments, you can navigate your healing journey with purpose and clarity, moving closer to your health and wellness aspirations.

Chapter 9: The Future of Self-Healing

The landscape of self-healing is rapidly evolving, driven by advancements in research and technology. As our understanding of the mind-body connection deepens, emerging research and innovations are paving the way for new approaches to health and wellness. This chapter explores the cutting-edge developments in self-healing, highlighting the potential of emerging research and technologies, as well as innovations in mind-body medicine, to transform our approach to health care.

Emerging Research and Technologies

The integration of technology into health care has led to the development of innovative tools and methodologies that enhance self-healing capabilities. From wearable devices that monitor vital signs in real-time to mobile apps that provide guided meditation and stress management techniques, technology is making it easier than ever to take an active role in our health.

- Wearable Health Technology: Devices like fitness trackers and smartwatches can track physical activity, sleep patterns, heart rate, and more, providing valuable data for personal health monitoring and improvement.
- Telehealth and Virtual Care: Telehealth platforms allow for remote consultations with healthcare providers, making it easier to access medical advice and mental health support from the comfort of home.
- Personalized Medicine: Advances in genomics and biotechnology are enabling more personalized approaches to health care, tailoring treatments and preventive strategies to the individual's genetic profile.
- AI and Machine Learning: Artificial intelligence (AI) and machine learning are being used to analyze health data, predict health outcomes, and develop personalized wellness plans, offering a new level of sophistication in self-care and disease prevention.

Innovations in Mind-Body Medicine

Mind-body medicine is experiencing a renaissance, with new research underscoring the profound impact of psychological and emotional factors on physical health. Innovative therapies and practices that harness this connection are gaining traction, offering promising avenues for self-healing.

- Biofeedback and Neurofeedback: These technologies provide real-time feedback on physiological processes, such as heart rate and brain activity, allowing individuals to learn how to consciously influence their physical state, improving stress management and emotional regulation.
- Virtual Reality (VR) Therapy: VR technology is being explored for therapeutic uses, including pain management, anxiety reduction, and the treatment of PTSD, by immersing patients in calming, controlled virtual environments.
- Mindfulness and Meditation Apps: A growing number of apps offer guided mindfulness and meditation exercises, making these practices more accessible and customizable, and supporting mental health and emotional well-being.

- Integrative Therapy Platforms: Platforms that combine various modalities of mind-body medicine, such as yoga, meditation, and cognitive-behavioral techniques, are becoming more common, offering holistic approaches to self-healing.

Conclusion

The future of self-healing is bright, with emerging research and technologies opening up new possibilities for improving health and well-being. As we continue to explore the interconnectedness of the mind and body, innovations in both technology and mind-body medicine hold the potential to revolutionize our approach to health care. By embracing these advancements, individuals can empower themselves to take control of their health, leading to a future where self-healing is an integral part of a comprehensive, personalized approach to wellness.

The Role of AI and Virtual Reality in Self-Healing

The integration of Artificial Intelligence (AI) and Virtual Reality (VR) into healthcare and wellness represents a significant leap forward in the field of self-healing. These technologies are not only expanding the boundaries of what's possible in medical treatment and therapy but are also offering innovative ways to support individual health and well-being. The role of AI and VR in self-healing encompasses a wide range of applications, from personalized health assessments and treatments to immersive therapeutic experiences.

AI in Self-Healing

AI's role in self-healing is multifaceted, offering advanced insights, personalization, and efficiency in health management. Key applications include:

- Personalized Health Recommendations: AI algorithms can analyze vast amounts of health data from wearable devices, electronic health records, and genetic tests to provide personalized health recommendations, optimizing individual wellness plans.
- Mental Health Support: AI-powered chatbots and mental health apps offer on-demand support, delivering cognitive behavioral therapy (CBT) techniques, mindfulness practices, and emotional support to users, making mental health care more accessible.
- Predictive Health Analytics: AI can predict potential health issues before they become serious, enabling preventive measures. For instance, AI can analyze patterns in heart rate variability to predict the risk of cardiovascular diseases, allowing for early intervention.

Virtual Reality in Self-Healing

VR technology offers immersive experiences that can significantly impact mental and physical health, including:

- Pain Management: VR has been used to manage chronic pain and during medical procedures to distract patients, reducing their perception of pain through immersive, calming environments or engaging activities.

- Stress Reduction and Relaxation: VR experiences can transport individuals to serene natural landscapes or guided meditations, promoting relaxation and stress reduction in a highly immersive way.
- Rehabilitation and Physical Therapy: VR applications in physical therapy allow patients to engage in virtual exercises tailored to their specific rehabilitation needs, making therapy more engaging and potentially more effective.
- Treatment of Phobias and Anxiety: Through controlled exposure in a safe, virtual environment, VR can be used to treat phobias, anxiety, and PTSD, allowing individuals to face their fears under the guidance of a therapist.

Conclusion

The roles of AI and VR in self-healing are emblematic of the exciting advancements at the intersection of technology and healthcare. By providing personalized health insights, accessible mental health support, immersive therapeutic experiences, and innovative rehabilitation tools, these technologies are significantly enhancing our ability to engage in self-healing practices. As AI and VR continue to evolve, their integration into healthcare promises to further empower individuals in their pursuit of health and well-being, making the future of self-healing more promising than ever.

The Role of Community and Social Support in Self-Healing

Community and social support play pivotal roles in the self-healing process, offering emotional sustenance, practical assistance, and a sense of belonging that can significantly influence health outcomes. The impact of social connections on health is well-documented, with research consistently showing that strong social ties can enhance well-being, increase longevity, and improve recovery rates from illness and surgery.

The Impact of Social Connections

Social connections—ranging from close familial bonds to broader community interactions—act as a buffer against the stressors of life, providing psychological and emotional support that is critical for maintaining mental and physical health.

- Emotional Support: The emotional support provided by friends, family, and community members can offer comfort, reduce stress, and foster a positive outlook, all of which are crucial for emotional and mental health.

- Practical Assistance: Social networks often provide practical help in times of need, such as assistance with daily tasks, care during illness, or financial support, which can alleviate stress and contribute to the healing process.

- Sense of Belonging: Being part of a community gives individuals a sense of belonging and identity, which is fundamental to psychological well-being. This sense of connection can motivate healthier lifestyle choices and adherence to treatment plans.

- Improved Mental Health: Social support is associated with lower rates of anxiety, depression, and loneliness. It can enhance self-esteem, provide a source of encouragement, and offer a platform for sharing experiences and coping strategies.

- Physical Health Benefits: Studies have shown that individuals with strong social networks tend to have better health outcomes, including lower risk of chronic diseases, higher rates of survival after a heart attack, and increased longevity. The stress-reducing effect of social support is a key factor in these health benefits.

Cultivating Social Connections for Self-Healing

- Engage with Community: Participate in community events, clubs, or groups that align with your interests. Volunteering can also be a rewarding way to connect with others and enhance your sense of purpose.

- Maintain and Strengthen Existing Relationships: Make an effort to sustain and deepen relationships with family and friends. Regular communication, shared activities, and mutual support strengthen these bonds.

- Seek Support Groups: For those dealing with specific health issues or life challenges, support groups can provide a sense of understanding, shared experience, and valuable coping strategies.

- Use Technology Wisely: While technology can help maintain connections, especially over long distances, prioritize face-to-face interactions when possible. Social media and online communities can complement but should not replace real-world interactions.

Conclusion

The role of community and social support in self-healing underscores the importance of social connections in overall health and well-being. By fostering strong relationships and engaging with a supportive community, individuals can enhance their resilience, reduce the impact of stress, and create a supportive environment conducive to healing and recovery. Recognizing the value of social support is essential in the journey towards holistic health, demonstrating that healing is not just a personal endeavor but a collective one as well.

Building a Supportive Network for Self-Healing

In the journey of self-healing, the importance of building a supportive network cannot be overstated. A strong support system can provide emotional encouragement, share valuable information, and offer practical assistance, all of which are crucial components for successful healing and personal growth. Whether you're navigating a health challenge, seeking to improve your well-being, or aiming to maintain a healthy lifestyle, the right network can significantly enhance your efforts.

Identifying Your Support Needs

Start by identifying what kind of support you need most. Support can be emotional, informational, or practical, and understanding your needs can help you seek out the right people and resources. Consider whether you need:

- Emotional Support: For empathy, understanding, and encouragement.
- Informational Support: For advice, knowledge, and sharing of experiences.
- Practical Support: For help with specific tasks or challenges.

Steps to Build Your Supportive Network

1. Leverage Existing Relationships:
   - Begin with family, friends, and colleagues who you feel comfortable sharing your self-healing journey with. Open communication about your goals and needs can deepen these relationships and make your support system more effective.

2. Connect with Healthcare Professionals:
   - Healthcare providers, therapists, and wellness coaches can offer professional guidance and support tailored to your health goals. Don't hesitate to ask questions and express your needs and preferences.

3. Join Support Groups and Communities:
   - Look for local or online support groups and communities focused on specific health conditions, wellness practices, or holistic health. These groups provide a platform to share experiences, learn from others, and find emotional and informational support.

4. Engage in Community Activities:
   - Participating in classes, workshops, or events related to your health interests (such as yoga, meditation, nutrition, etc.) can connect you with like-minded individuals and experts in the field.

5. Utilize Online Resources:
   - Online forums, social media groups, and health and wellness blogs and websites can be valuable resources for information and support. However, ensure the sources are reputable and the advice is evidence-based.

6. Volunteer or Offer Support to Others:
   - Offering support to others can not only help them but also strengthen your own sense of purpose and connection. Volunteering in health-related organizations or groups can expand your network and foster meaningful relationships.

Nurturing Your Support Network

Building a support network is an ongoing process. Nurturing these relationships involves regular communication, mutual respect, and gratitude. Be open to both giving and receiving support, and recognize that the needs and dynamics of your support network may change over time.

Conclusion

A supportive network is an invaluable asset in the self-healing journey, offering emotional comfort, shared knowledge, and practical assistance. By actively building and nurturing this network, you can enhance your resilience, motivation, and capacity for healing. Remember, the journey of health and wellness is not one you have to undertake alone; through the strength of community and connection, you can navigate the path of self-healing with greater confidence and support.

Personal Stories of Transformation

Inspiring Examples

Personal stories of transformation can serve as powerful sources of inspiration and insight for those on their own journey of self-healing and personal growth. These narratives not only highlight the resilience of the human spirit but also illustrate the diverse paths and strategies individuals have employed to overcome challenges and achieve significant positive changes in their lives. Here are examples of personal transformation stories that inspire and offer valuable lessons.

Overcoming Health Challenges

John's Story: After being diagnosed with type 2 diabetes, John faced the reality of his unhealthy lifestyle. Instead of relying solely on medication, he embarked on a comprehensive self-healing journey that included a plant-based diet, regular exercise, and mindfulness practices. Over the course of a year, not only did John significantly reduce his blood sugar levels, but he also lost weight, gained energy, and improved his overall well-being. John's story demonstrates the power of lifestyle changes in managing chronic health conditions.

Transforming Through Mindfulness and Meditation

Sara's Story: Struggling with anxiety and depression for years, Sara found her turning point when she began practicing mindfulness and meditation. These practices helped her develop greater emotional awareness and resilience, leading to profound changes in how she managed stress and approached life's challenges. Sara's journey highlights the transformative potential of mindfulness and meditation in improving mental health and quality of life.

Achieving Personal Growth Through Adversity

Alex's Story: After a serious accident left Alex with chronic pain and mobility issues, they faced the prospect of a drastically altered life. Through a combination of physical therapy, yoga, and joining a support group for individuals with similar injuries, Alex not only regained much of their physical strength but also discovered a new passion for helping others. Alex's story illustrates how adversity can lead to personal growth, new directions, and a deepened sense of purpose.

Lifestyle Transformation for Holistic Well-being

Maya's Story: Maya, a high-powered executive, experienced a wake-up call regarding her health and happiness after suffering from burnout. She decided to prioritize her well-being by adopting a holistic lifestyle, incorporating balanced nutrition, regular physical activity, and practices for mental and emotional health, such as journaling and spending time in nature. Maya's transformation shows the importance of balance and holistic self-care in achieving sustainable well-being.

From Isolation to Community and Connection

Kevin's Story: Feeling isolated and disconnected, Kevin struggled with social anxiety and a sense of loneliness. His journey to transformation began when he volunteered at a local community center, where he found not only a sense of belonging but also the courage to share his experiences and support others. Kevin's story underscores the healing power of community and the positive impact of reaching out and connecting with others.

Conclusion

These personal stories of transformation offer a glimpse into the myriad ways individuals can navigate their healing journeys, overcome obstacles, and achieve meaningful change. They remind us of the importance of resilience, the potential for growth in the face of adversity, and the transformative power of adopting holistic approaches to health and well-being. By sharing and reflecting on these stories, we can find motivation, hope, and guidance on our own paths to wellness and personal growth.

Lessons Learned: Insights from Personal Transformation Stories

The journey of self-healing and personal transformation, as illustrated by the inspiring examples shared, offers profound lessons that can guide others in their pursuit of health, well-being, and personal growth. These narratives not only showcase the resilience and resourcefulness of individuals facing various challenges but also highlight key insights and strategies that can be applied more broadly. Here are some of the essential lessons learned from these stories of transformation:

1. The Power of Holistic Approaches

- Insight: Addressing both the physical and emotional aspects of well-being is crucial for sustainable healing and growth. Integrating practices that nurture the body, mind, and spirit leads to more comprehensive and lasting changes.
- Application: Consider all facets of your well-being in your healing plan. Combine physical activities with mental health practices such as mindfulness or counseling for a balanced approach.

2. The Importance of Personal Agency and Responsibility

- Insight: Taking an active role in one's healing journey empowers individuals to make meaningful changes and achieve their health goals. Personal agency involves making informed choices and taking responsibility for those choices.
- Application: Educate yourself about your health conditions and treatment options. Be proactive in making lifestyle changes and seeking out resources that support your goals.

3. Adaptability and Openness to Change

- Insight: Healing often requires adapting to new circumstances and being open to changing long-standing habits and behaviors. Flexibility in the face of challenges is a key factor in successful transformation.
- Application: Be willing to adjust your strategies and plans as you progress. Stay open to new information and alternative approaches that may enhance your journey.

4. The Role of Support and Community

- Insight: A supportive network of friends, family, healthcare providers, and even peers facing similar challenges can provide encouragement, advice, and a sense of belonging. Community support is invaluable for navigating the ups and downs of the healing process.
- Application: Seek out and nurture supportive relationships. Consider joining groups or communities that align with your healing journey.

5. Resilience and Perseverance

- Insight: Overcoming obstacles and setbacks is often part of the healing journey. Resilience—the ability to bounce back from difficulties—combined with perseverance, is crucial for achieving long-term goals.
- Application: Develop coping strategies that bolster your resilience. Celebrate small victories along the way, and maintain focus on your larger objectives.

6. Mindfulness and Self-awareness

- Insight: Cultivating mindfulness and self-awareness enhances emotional regulation and stress management, contributing significantly to mental and emotional well-being.
- Application: Practice mindfulness or other meditative techniques regularly. Engage in reflective practices, such as journaling, to increase self-awareness.

7. The Significance of Self-compassion

- Insight: Healing is a journey, not a destination. Practicing self-compassion—being kind and understanding toward oneself in the face of challenges—is essential for maintaining motivation and emotional health.
- Application: Treat yourself with kindness and understanding, especially during difficult times. Recognize that setbacks are part of the process and offer opportunities for growth.

Conclusion

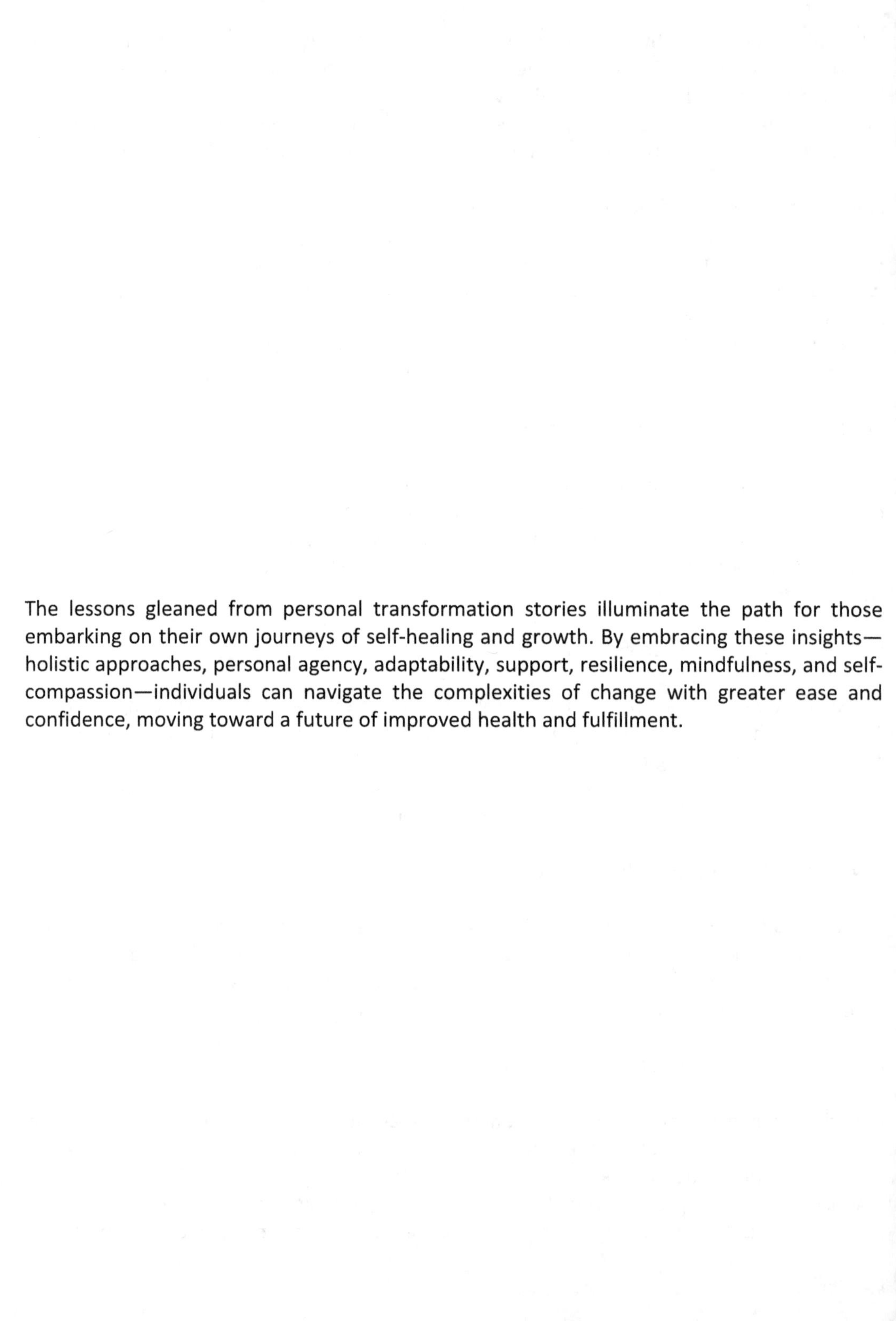

The lessons gleaned from personal transformation stories illuminate the path for those embarking on their own journeys of self-healing and growth. By embracing these insights—holistic approaches, personal agency, adaptability, support, resilience, mindfulness, and self-compassion—individuals can navigate the complexities of change with greater ease and confidence, moving toward a future of improved health and fulfillment.

Conclusion

The Ongoing Journey of Self-Healing and Embracing a Holistic View

The journey of self-healing is a profound and ongoing process that extends beyond the resolution of physical symptoms or the attainment of specific health goals. It encompasses a continuous exploration and nurturing of one's physical, emotional, mental, and spiritual well-being. Embracing a holistic view of health recognizes that these aspects of the self are deeply interconnected, influencing one another in complex and significant ways. As we conclude, it's important to reflect on the essence of this journey and the holistic perspective that guides it.

The Ongoing Journey of Self-Healing

Self-healing is not a linear path but a cyclical process of growth, learning, and adaptation. It involves periods of progress, as well as challenges and setbacks, each offering valuable lessons and opportunities for deeper understanding and transformation. The journey is characterized by:

- Self-discovery: Continually learning about one's body, mind, and emotional landscape, uncovering new insights into personal health and well-being.
- Self-care: Actively engaging in practices that support and nourish all aspects of one's health, from nutrition and exercise to stress management and emotional expression.
- Self-compassion: Approaching oneself with kindness, understanding, and patience, recognizing that healing is a process that requires time, effort, and forgiveness.

Embracing a Holistic View

A holistic approach to self-healing emphasizes the integration of various dimensions of health and well-being. It advocates for:

- Balance: Seeking harmony between different areas of life—work, relationships, leisure, and self-care—to support overall health.
- Connection: Recognizing the impact of social relationships, community, and environmental factors on health and actively fostering positive connections.
- Personalization: Tailoring health strategies to fit individual needs, preferences, and circumstances, acknowledging that there is no one-size-fits-all solution to health and healing.

Moving Forward

As individuals continue on their self-healing journey, embracing a holistic view encourages a broader perspective on health—one that transcends physical symptoms and seeks to cultivate a life of balance, fulfillment, and well-being. This approach invites an ongoing commitment to:

- Learning and Growth: Remaining open to new knowledge, experiences, and practices that can support health and personal development.

- Adaptability: Being willing to adjust and refine one's approach to health and healing as needs and circumstances change.
- Empowerment: Taking an active role in one's health journey, making informed choices, and advocating for one's well-being.

Conclusion

The journey of self-healing is a dynamic and lifelong pursuit, enriched by a holistic view of health that integrates the physical, emotional, mental, and spiritual dimensions of the self. By embracing this comprehensive approach, individuals can navigate the complexities of health and well-being with resilience, purpose, and joy. As we move forward, let us carry the lessons learned, the insights gained, and the connections fostered, continuing to explore, heal, and grow in all aspects of our lives.

Next Steps for Readers: Embarking on Your Self-Healing Journey

As you conclude this exploration of self-healing and holistic well-being, you are equipped with insights, strategies, and inspirational examples to guide you on your journey. The path forward involves integrating what you've learned into daily life and taking proactive steps toward health and fulfillment. Here are actionable next steps for readers ready to embark on or continue their self-healing journey:

1. Reflect and Assess

- Take time to reflect on your current health and well-being. Assess your physical, emotional, mental, and spiritual health to identify areas you wish to improve or focus on.

2. Set Personal Goals

- Based on your assessment, set clear, achievable goals for your health and well-being. Use the SMART criteria to ensure your goals are Specific, Measurable, Achievable, Relevant, and Time-bound.

3. Create a Holistic Plan

- Develop a holistic plan that addresses various aspects of your health. Incorporate elements like nutrition, exercise, stress management, and activities that foster emotional and spiritual well-being.

4. Gather Resources and Support

- Identify resources and support systems that can aid your journey. This might include books, websites, healthcare professionals, support groups, and community resources.

5. Implement and Experiment

- Begin implementing your plan, but remain open to experimentation. Be willing to try different approaches to find what works best for you.

6. Track Progress and Adjust

- Keep a journal or use digital tools to track your progress towards your goals. Reflect on what's working and what isn't, and be prepared to adjust your plan as needed.

7. Practice Self-compassion and Patience

- Approach your journey with kindness and patience. Healing and growth are processes that take time, and self-compassion is a key component of sustainable change.

8. Stay Informed and Open

- Continue to educate yourself on aspects of self-healing and holistic health. Stay open to new information, perspectives, and practices that can enhance your journey.

9. Share and Connect

- Share your experiences and insights with others. Connecting with individuals on similar paths can provide mutual support, inspiration, and a sense of community.

10. Celebrate Your Achievements

- Take time to celebrate your achievements, no matter how small. Recognizing your progress can provide motivation and affirm the value of your efforts.

Conclusion

Your journey of self-healing and personal growth is uniquely yours, marked by individual choices, experiences, and discoveries. By taking these next steps, you actively engage in shaping your path toward health and well-being. Remember, the journey is ongoing, filled with opportunities for learning, healing, and transformation. Embrace it with curiosity, openness, and a commitment to your holistic health, and watch as your life unfolds in more vibrant and fulfilling ways.

Appendices

Appendix A: Resources for Further Reading

1. "The Body Keeps the Score: Brain, Mind, and Body in the Healing of Trauma" by Bessel van der Kolk
   - An exploration of how trauma affects the body and mind, and innovative paths to recovery.

2. "How to Heal Yourself When No One Else Can: A Total Self-Healing Approach for Mind, Body, and Spirit" by Amy B. Scher
   - A guide to self-healing techniques that address the whole person for comprehensive healing.

3. "Mind Over Medicine: Scientific Proof That You Can Heal Yourself" by Lissa Rankin, M.D.
   - An examination of the medical evidence supporting the body's ability to heal itself, and how to utilize this power.

4. "The Healing Self: A Revolutionary New Plan to Supercharge Your Immunity and Stay Well for Life" by Deepak Chopra and Rudolph E. Tanzi
   - Insights into the body's potential for self-repair and how lifestyle choices can boost health and longevity.

5. "Full Catastrophe Living: Using the Wisdom of Your Body and Mind to Face Stress, Pain, and Illness" by Jon Kabat-Zinn
   - A comprehensive guide to using mindfulness meditation as a tool for dealing with stress, pain, and illness.

Appendix B: Guide to Meditation and Mindfulness Apps

1. Headspace
   - Offers guided meditations, sleep sounds, and mindfulness exercises designed for all levels.

2. Calm
   - Features a wide range of meditation options, sleep stories, and music tracks to reduce anxiety and improve sleep.

3. Insight Timer
   - A free app with thousands of guided meditations and courses on a wide array of topics from mindfulness to stress reduction.

4. 10% Happier
   - Provides practical, accessible meditations and teachings for fending off stress and living a happier life.

5. MyLife Meditation (formerly Stop, Breathe & Think)

- Encourages users to check in with their emotions and offers personalized meditation and mindfulness experiences.

Appendix C: Directory of Professional Help

1. Psychology Today Therapist Directory
   - An online directory to find therapists, psychiatrists, therapy groups, and wellness professionals near you.

2. National Center for Complementary and Integrative Health (NCCIH)
   - Provides information on finding healthcare providers who specialize in complementary and integrative health practices.

3. American Association of Naturopathic Physicians (AANP)
   - Offers a directory of licensed naturopathic doctors who are trained in holistic and natural approaches to medicine.

4. International Association of Yoga Therapists (IAYT)
   - A resource for finding certified yoga therapists who use yoga practices to address health issues and promote well-being.

5. American Massage Therapy Association (AMTA)
   - Features a locator service to find qualified massage therapists across the United States.

Conclusion

These appendices provide a starting point for readers seeking to deepen their understanding of self-healing, explore mindfulness and meditation practices, or connect with professional help tailored to their needs. Embracing these resources can enhance your journey toward health and well-being, offering guidance, support, and inspiration along the way.

Glossary

Acupuncture: A traditional Chinese medicine technique involving the insertion of needles into specific points on the body to alleviate pain and treat various health conditions.

Biofeedback: A technique that uses electronic monitoring to convey information about physiological processes, enabling an individual to gain control over bodily functions.

Chronic Pain: Long-standing pain that persists beyond the usual course of an acute illness or healing of an injury, often without a clear cause.

Cognitive Behavioral Therapy (CBT): A psychotherapeutic approach that addresses dysfunctional emotions, behaviors, and cognitions through a goal-oriented, systematic process.

Holistic Health: An approach to life that considers the whole person and how he or she interacts with their environment, emphasizing the connection of mind, body, and spirit.

Integrative Medicine: A healing-oriented medicine that takes into account the whole person, including all aspects of lifestyle, and emphasizes the therapeutic relationship between practitioner and patient.

Meditation: A practice where an individual uses a technique – such as mindfulness, or focusing the mind on a particular object, thought, or activity – to train attention and awareness, and achieve a mentally clear and emotionally calm and stable state.

Mind-Body Connection: The theory that the mind and body are not separate entities but interlinked, and that psychological well-being can affect physical health and vice versa.

Mindfulness: The practice of being fully present and engaged in the moment, aware of one's thoughts and feelings without distraction or judgment.

Neurofeedback: A type of biofeedback that uses real-time displays of brain activity—most commonly electroencephalography (EEG)—to teach self-regulation of brain function.

Qi (Chi): In traditional Chinese culture, Qi is believed to be a vital force forming part of any living entity. Qi translates as "air" and figuratively as "material energy," "life force," or "energy flow."

Self-Healing: The process by which an individual facilitates the recovery of health and well-being through innate, personal power and action, often involving holistic or alternative practices.

Yoga: A group of physical, mental, and spiritual practices or disciplines that originated in ancient India, aimed at controlling the mind, body, and soul to achieve a state of peace and liberation.

References

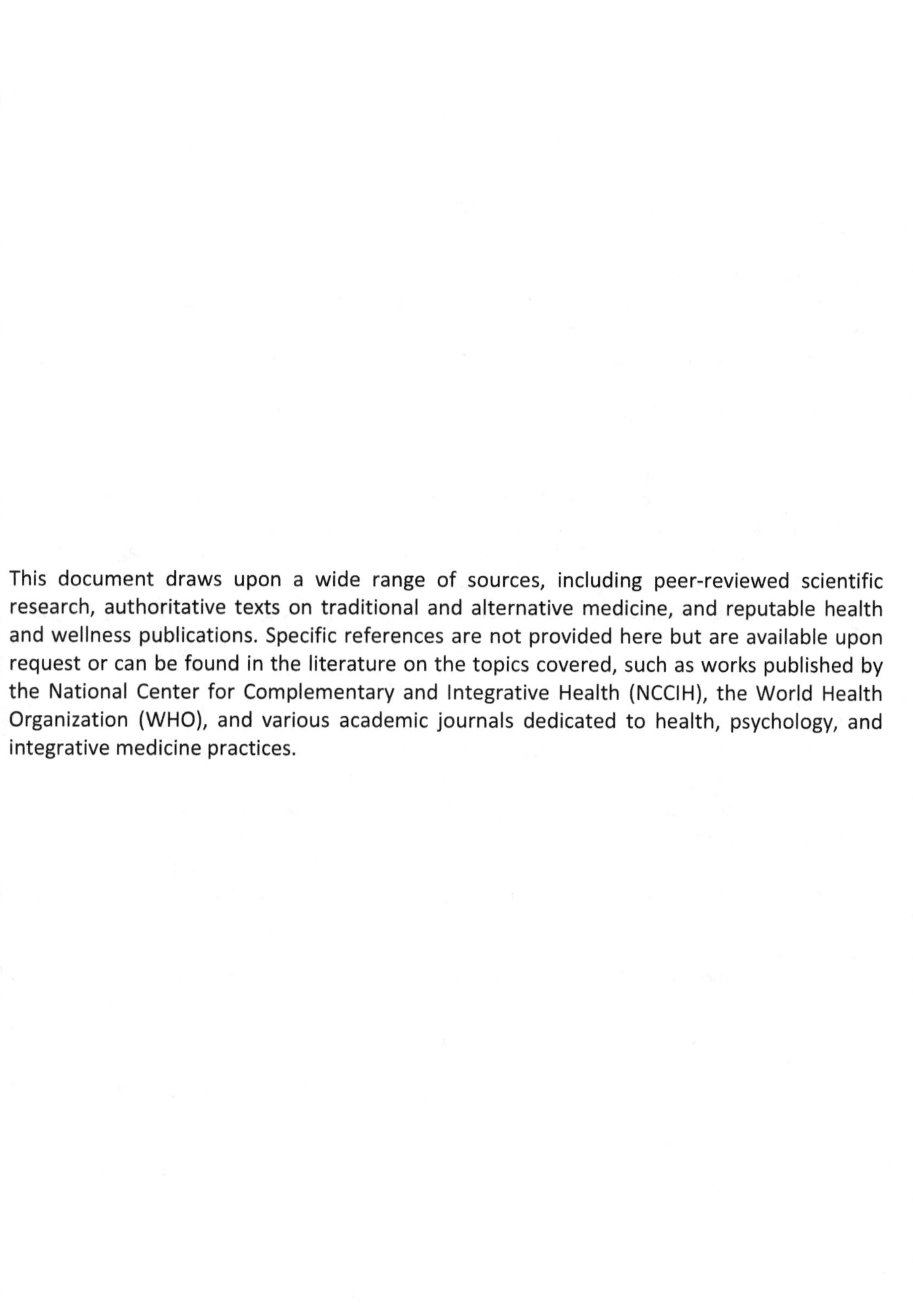

This document draws upon a wide range of sources, including peer-reviewed scientific research, authoritative texts on traditional and alternative medicine, and reputable health and wellness publications. Specific references are not provided here but are available upon request or can be found in the literature on the topics covered, such as works published by the National Center for Complementary and Integrative Health (NCCIH), the World Health Organization (WHO), and various academic journals dedicated to health, psychology, and integrative medicine practices.

References for further reading

Academic Journals
- Journal of Alternative and Complementary Medicine: Research on alternative and complementary medicine practices.
- Mindfulness: Studies and articles on the practice and effects of mindfulness and meditation.
- Pain Medicine: Research on pain management, including non-pharmacological approaches.

Books and Authoritative Texts
- "The Body Keeps the Score: Brain, Mind, and Body in the Healing of Trauma" by Bessel van der Kolk: Insight into how trauma impacts health and methods for recovery.
- "Mind Over Medicine: Scientific Proof That You Can Heal Yourself" by Lissa Rankin, M.D.: Exploration of the body's self-healing potential and how to harness it.
- "Full Catastrophe Living: Using the Wisdom of Your Body and Mind to Face Stress, Pain, and Illness" by Jon Kabat-Zinn: A guide to using mindfulness meditation for health and well-being.

Online Resources
- PubMed Central (PMC): A free archive of biomedical and life sciences journal literature at the U.S. National Institutes of Health's National Library of Medicine.
- National Center for Complementary and Integrative Health (NCCIH): Government-sponsored resources on complementary and integrative health practices.
- World Health Organization (WHO): Reports and guidelines on various health topics, including traditional, complementary, and integrative health approaches.

Professional Organizations
- American Psychological Association (APA): Resources on psychological well-being and mental health treatments.
- International Association of Yoga Therapists (IAYT): Publications and research on yoga as a therapeutic practice.
- American Massage Therapy Association (AMTA): Evidence and guidelines on the benefits of massage therapy.